Brazil's

SOULFUL

MEDICINE

ISBN 0-7414-4299-X

Published by:

INFINITY
PUBLISHING.COM

1094 New DeHaven Street, Suite 100
West Conshohocken, PA 19428-2713
Info@buybooksontheweb.com
www.buybooksontheweb.com
Toll-free (877) BUY BOOK
Local Phone (610) 941-9999
Fax (610) 941-9959

Printed in the United States of America

Printed on Recycled Paper

Published September 2008

DEDICATION AND ACKNOWLEDGMENTS

Never had I embarked on a journey that would take me to discover a new field of scientific spirituality, as Brazil has come to offer. With each trip to Brazil since my first in December 2001, I have been exposed to the greater realms of medicine, one engulfed in light, or rather in illuminating intelligence; in a service of love, and compassion. Brazil has shown exceptional human qualities, particularly in the solidarity it reaches beyond its borders.

I owe this book to my husband Joe, for all his encouragement and support. I dedicate this book to you for your selflessness, your service to Love. To my children and grandchildren I thank you for believing in me and encouraging me to bring this book to fruition. To the fondest memory of my *abuelita* (my maternal grandmother), I thank her for teaching me the value of faith, hope, prayer, and humility.

I would also like to thank our adopted Brazilian family, *familia* Oliveira, from Salvador, Bahia for introducing us to the beautiful Brazilian culture and, for sharing their wonderful spiritual insight and hospitality with my family and I. To *familia* Pimentel of Cruz Alta and Porto Alegre, Brazil, I thank you for your warm hospitality and friendship during the research involved in this book. To our extended spiritual family of Abadiania, Brazil, thank you for your constant prayers and support. To our spiritual brother Juan Tobias Leon, I am indebted to you for introducing the wondrous works of João de Deus and the Casa de Dom Inácio, in Abadiania, Brazil.

To my mentors Dr. Jeanette Castellanos, for believing in me and for your selfless service to all of your students, "*gracias;*" and to Professor Melvin Aaron, who instilled in me a genuine desire for the pursuit of justice, and truth, for this I remain eternally grateful to you. To all my professors whom contributed in some form to this work, thank you for sharing your wisdom, vision, and willingness to help make this planet a better place for everyone, you know who you are. May God Bless each one of you.

To all genuine healers, educators, scientists, health practitioners, theologians, and philosophers who dedicate themselves selflessly to the advancement of the human race while embracing peace, and solidarity, thank you for your invaluable collaboration and service.

To all those involved in the monumental task of the progress of humanity. May the Light of the Creator continue to light your paths in the re-creation of the planet.

Lastly, I dedicate this work to the loving memory of my brother Ricardo, and my cousin Magda. May the peace, brotherhood and sisterhood I have found in Brazil be heartfelt by them in the spirit world.

CONTENTS

INTRODUCTION i

Science and Mysticism are Different Paths, But the Same Truth i

I. A BRAZILIAN HEALTH OVERVIEW 1

1. A BRIEF HISTORY OF THE ORIGINS OF BRAZILIAN SPIRITUAL HEALING 3
2. SPIRIT HEALING WITHIN THE CONTEXT OF OTHER HEALING SYSTEMS AND BIOMEDICINE 13
3. THE SCIENTIFIC, PHILOSOPHICAL, AND MORAL ASPECTS OF BRAZILIAN MEDICINE 23

II. MAXIMIZING SPIRIT MEDICINE 33

4. CONCEPTS OF THE BRAZILIAN SPIRITUAL WORLDVIEW 35
5. THE RELATIONSHIP BETWEEN SOUL, MIND, BODY, HEALTH AND ILLNESS 45
6. THE HUMAN ENERGY SYSTEM AND THE ROLE OF EMOTIONS IN HEALTH 51

III. SOUL DOCTORS, SOUL CLINICS, AND SOUL TREATMENT 57

7. SOUL DOCTORS, SOUL CLINICS: THE SACRED MISSION OF HEALING MEDIUMS 59

8. ABADIANIA'S HEALING PHENOMENON: JOÃO DE DEUS 63

9. CASA DE DOM INÁCIO: A MULTI-FAITH NON-DENOMINATIONAL HEALING SANCTUARY: TREATS WOUNDED AND FLABBY SOULS 69

10. PATRON ENTITY OF THE CASA DE DOM INÁCIO: SAINT IGNATIUS DE LOYOLA 77

11. NON-SURGICAL TREATMENT MODALITIES AND REGIMENS 85

12. SPIRITUAL SURGERIES 105

IV. CHANGING THE MODEL TO INCLUDE MORAL AND SOCIAL HEALTH 115

13. HUMANISTIC MEDICINE INVOLVES AN INTEGRATIVE APPROACH: WHY OUTDATED MODELS MUST CHANGE 117

14. BUILDING NEW HEALTH PARTNERSHIPS WHILE IMPROVING SOCIAL CONDITIONS: TRABALHANDO 125

15. FINAL THOUGHTS 133

BRAZILIAN AND UNIVERSAL PRAYERS 137

GLOSSARY 165

READINGS FOR FURTHER STUDY 195

BIBLIOGRAPHY 201

ABOUT THE AUTHOR 205

FOR JOE
AND ALL THOSE HELPING TO UPLIFT HUMANITY

INTRODUCTION

SCIENCE AND MYSTICISM ARE DIFFERENT PATHS, BUT THE SAME TRUTH

Brazil is typically not associated with Latin American culture because of a language difference with it's Latin American neighbors. Colonized by Portugal, Brazil naturally adapted Portuguese as its official language. With the exception of language however, Brazil and Spanish Latin America share other historical and cultural similaritics: European colonization, a native indigenous culture, and a history of slavery, African ancestry, and an important spiritual legacy. Brazil considered by its people to be the heart and soul of the world, believes it will lead the world in its healing and spiritual evolution.

Contained in this work is a presentation of the unique combination of scientific and supernatural knowledge utilized in Brazilian spiritual healing and psychic surgical practices, within the context of the world's spiritual and scientific evolution. This unique

Brazilian medical repertoire provides the patient with a practical path of self-discovery, personal transformation, and self-responsibility.

Spiritual healing intervenes at the conscious plane, and provides appropriate behavioral guidelines that are capable of freeing the patient's soul from obstructions, which could otherwise lead to disease and/or suffering. It is the moral teachings contained in the Christian Gospel that constitute principles concerning behavior in all instances of private and public life, having a direct impact on the individual's health.

In it's spiritual quest to lead the world in the humanization of medicine, Brazilians have come to be great educators who already are working on the construction of an integrative model of health. Brazilian spirituality, it's major concepts, teachings, history, and how Brazilians have utilized it for healing will be the highlight of this major multi-disciplinary effort.

Included will be a description of the spiritual diagnostic and treatment protocols, the spiritual surgical procedures, and an explanation of how these actively promote healing. A presentation of the scientific, philosophical, and moral aspects of Brazilian spiritual healing will be followed by a practical discussion, based on a medical and humanistic perspective, of the need for cooperation between science and religion.

Professional as well as individual patient experiences involving Brazilian spiritual healing along with other medical and spiritual knowledge found in ancient traditions, can when analyzed critically and in depth, offer a greater understanding of what makes a healthcare delivery system more effective and efficient; provide genuine integral health; and focus on prevention-oriented (as opposed to maintenance-oriented) healthcare, while also maintaining costs, and integrity that does not sacrifice quality or treatment outcomes.

Although this form of unorthodox healing may initially not "digest well," this information will definitely challenge some established common-sense assumptions of the world, in particular as these apply to biomedicine and what most perceive as the *only* "real knowledge." Even when empirical observation and facts are presented, such information may still be difficult to accept because comprehending it may contradict individual secular teachings and/or religious upbringing.

The goal of the author is to present valuable information objectively in order to analyze it in its most critical form, without directly or indirectly discrediting any related educational, scientific, medical, or religious institution or individual. The objective of this work is to provide insight to some of the many misconceptions about spiritual/psychic healing and surgical practices within the larger context of medical science, philosophy and morality. Bringing forth the ideological foundations found in these three disciplines is essential. They are the integral components behind a collaborative global working relationship between humanity's spiritual and healing traditions and biomedicine.

Spiritual healing has a deep connection to the human soul. Its diagnosis and treatment cannot be dealt with by classic medicine alone, as it does not yet have the required knowledge, preparation or training to adequately understand, formulate, and implement a required transcendental model of health. Principles that have been validated by facts and observations that have derived from all academic disciplines, and collected in different parts of the world, warrant consideration.

In acknowledging and humbling itself to other important aspects of the human experience, and incorporating these into the current medical paradigm, biomedicine as well as humanity in general would have finally met a most important evolutionary objective.

Only by answering deep philosophical questions with physical measurements, as Brazilians are now undertaking, will humanity be able to transcend into a new medical paradigm that more adequately fits the unique needs of the individual. Brazilian spiritual healing is getting humanity closer to understanding the most fundamental truths governing the human body and the laws of the universe.

PART ONE

A BRAZILIAN HEALTH OVERVIEW

1

A BRIEF HISTORY OF THE ORIGINS OF BRAZILIAN SPIRITUAL HEALING

The idea of spirits influencing thoughts, actions, health and illness was not born of the Spiritist doctrine nor was it born in Brazil. It has existed since early human life on earth. All religions preach in a direct or indirect way about the existence of a spiritual world. None completely deny these spiritual interventions. Throughout time, many religious institutions have created dogmas, and ceremonial rituals related to this universal belief of the spirit world.

Still today it is not uncommon to find the faithful praying in fellowship with a spirit entity (such as angels, saints or benevolent spirits), in asking them to take their prayer petition before their Creator, or to simply second their petition. It is not unusual in today's modern times for exorcisms to take place [exorcisms are done to either curb the power of the devil and prevent him from doing harm, or to expel evil spirits from a possessed person]. Only from a historical perspective can Brazil's mediumistic medicine be more completely assessed and appreciated.

Native American Indians of Brazil, the Tupinamba, had certainly suffered from illness prior to the arrival of the Europeans. They counted however, on the village shaman to intercede for their good fortune and health. Gifted with specialized universal, esoteric, and empirical knowledge and being aware of universal cosmic rules concerning calendrical matters, agriculture, weather, horticulture, astronomy and cosmology, shamans were allowed to harness the forces of nature in order to meet the health and survival needs of his people.

It is evident that European medicine did nothing for the native population. For the village shaman who had succumbed to the European priests conversion efforts, the harmony and future of his community had forever been altered. Concerned with the successful conversion of pagans, priests and the church saw in these supernaturally powerful men a significant threat to their conversion efforts and decided they would have to strip them of their power.

In their efforts to convert "heathens" to "people of reason," European friars reduced the shamanic healing tradition to one that was characterized as non-reputable, ignorant, and incompetent. This left the sole supernatural power in the hands of the priest, now the principal intermediary between the physical and the superior spiritual spheres. Interestingly, however, friars did not hesitate to learn from the indigenous advanced ethno-botanical knowledge, which exerted great influence on the developing European pharmacopoeia.

By 1530 African slaves arrived in Bahia, in northeast Brazil, bringing their own healing medicine and magic. African healers, their knowledge, and a belief system strongly influenced by stories of "*orixás*" (spirits), soon adapted to the indigenous and European healing traditions.

But once baptized as Christians, as had previously occurred with the indigenous peoples of the new world, African slaves creatively adopted the Christian spirits and combined them with their own *orixás*. "Olorun, god of creation was thought of as God the Father, or Jehova. Obatalá, god of the heavens and purity, merged with Jesus Christ. His daughter, Yemanjá, merged with the Virgin Mary," and her children with various other Christian saints, notes Krippner (1987, pp. 274-275). He adds, "there was no direct counterpart for Satan in Yoruba mythology. The closest that could be derived were the *ifás* and the *exus,* messengers of the gods and guardians of the temples who were quite mischievous, sometimes mixing up people's prayers and granting them someone else's request" (p. 275). Spirits were considered to be very important in healing ceremonies.

African based medicine was received with a greater contempt than that of the indigenous peoples of Brazil. The African worldview, as seen by Portuguese and Spanish colonists was one that was more deeply submerged in idolatry, superstition, and allegiance to supernatural powers, than its indigenous counterpart. Africans dominion over supernatural powers extended into prevention and removal of spells, as well as white magic. The idea of African magic and medicine in Brazil came to be known as a type of deviant science, going as far as to prohibit African slaves the use of plants for medicine or surgery. Even to consult a slave on any medical issue was banned.

While the pre-colonial Portuguese worldview undoubtedly included the existence of mystical forces, the church, as far as it was concerned, considered these mundane activities to be neither good nor bad, they were morally neutral. Supernatural activities, such as love potions, amulets, and divination, were used for specific ends; were not negatively viewed nor considered dangerous. It was only in the centuries that followed colonization that Christianity redefined magic and supernatural powers as the handiwork of Satan (Voeks).

African slaves realizing their inferior position in the new world, perceived European magic as far more powerful than their own. That they were slaves and the Europeans were masters was enough proof that Europeans too had control of supernatural forces. Rather than to relinquish their practices, slaves adopted the European healing repertoire. This syncretism gave the Afro-Brazilian practitioner a new position of considerable status and power among his people as well as among the ruling class. The role of folk healer, herbalist, diviner, and shaman, as well as that of magician and sorcerer – which had long been vacated by the demise of the Tupinamba – would come to be occupied by *pais and mães-de-santo*, Afro-Brazilian priests and priestesses of the Yoruba religion known as *Candomblé*, the religion of the *orixás.* This syncretism among the indigenous, African, and Catholic religions occurred effortlessly as they all had great similarities (Voeks).

The Yoruba belief that transcendental communication is a means to an end continued on with *Candomblé* in the state of Bahia and is found in many other religious ceremonies and rituals. Notes Voeks (1997), "The cosmologies of both religions are essentially pantheistic; both recognize a high god, distant and largely inaccessible to mortals, as well as a pantheon of lesser divinities, to whom direct appeal can be made during periods of adversity. Like the Yoruba Gods and goddesses, who are viewed as deified heroes of African antiquity, the Catholic saints once were mortal beings, whose exceptional deeds are immortalized in myth. And, like their West African counterparts, the saints took on certain qualities: dominion over nature, control of fertility, and influence over health" (Pp. 59-60).

From the fertile grounds of the *Candomblé* spirit tradition, a new influence came almost three centuries later with Allan Kardec's *Book of Spirits*. Making its debut in Brazil in 1875, this book written in France, was channeled from spirit; it has helped establish important principles of communication between the physical and spiritual worlds. This work stresses the need for inner transformation and self-knowledge as avenues to fulfillment and personal realization on earth. It is considered a classic of spiritual literature (translated to forty-five languages).

Kardec's other books, among them, *The Gospel According to Spiritism* helped redefine concepts of human suffering, imperfection, and disease for many Brazilians. *"Kardecismo"* offered a new therapeutic regimen. A new life based on a systematic study of illuminating *spiritual and scientific texts* offered a promising evolutionary path to one's greater self.

By the end of the 19th century, Spiritism (aka Kardecism) and the deep-seated Homeopathic movement in Brazil brought from Germany, would prove to be the impetus to the next Brazilian phenomenon, the spiritist-healing movement. The humanization of medicine in Brazil was accomplished through the selfless works of Dr. Adolfo Bezerra de Menezes. After studying philosophy and the Spiritist doctrine, Menezes immediately identified with the spiritual knowledge of Kardec's books, becoming a devout defender of the gospel teachings of Christ. He was a most influential figure in the spiritist-healing movement, as well as other social movements of the time. He is known as the *Doctor of the Poor, the Brazilian Kardec*, spending his entire life fighting for many human causes – the human rights of the poor, as well as for the right and freedom of both slaves and spiritists.

As Brazil's most consciously active, and vocal figure of the 19th century, Bezerra de Menezes erected a multitude of spiritist centers and communities throughout Brazil, and in 1888 he became the president of the Brazilian Spiritist Federation. He served poor patients without ever expecting or receiving any form of payment. Even after his passing he has remained a type of folk saint among Brazilians of all classes. Many believe his benevolent spirit continues to work from the spirit realm through mediumistic healers, such as João de Deus at the Casa de Dom Inácio in Abadiania, Brazil.

By the turn of the 20th Century (1904), other spiritist groups much like *Candomblé* were founded in Rio de Janeiro, *Macumba* and *Umbanda*, also emphasizing the importance of spirit incorporation in healing ceremonies, venerating Jesus Christ and using Christian names rather than the African appellations. While all three major spiritist groups differ in the ceremonial and ritualistic aspect (*Kardecismo* is ritual free), they hold several beliefs in common: "(1) humans have a physical body and a spiritual body; (2) discarnate spirits are in constant contact with the physical world; (3) humans can learn how to incorporate spirit guides for the purpose of healing" (Krippner, 1987, p. 276). These three major syncretic groupings, *Candomblé, Kardecismo, and Umbanda*, have helped shape an integral part of the Brazilian spiritual mindset, as they know it today. While these groups are responsible for much of the Brazilian ideology, the importance of Catholicism in this country cannot go without mention.

The population of Roman Catholics in Brazil is the largest in the world. In 2003 approximately 79% of the population (approximately 125 million) were Catholics. Today the formation of a strong Christian and fraternal character that symbolizes most Brazilians is predominantly due to more than 400 years of Catholicism, brought to Brazil during the Church's conversion efforts.

Francisco Cândido Xavier, a world renown medium from Uberaba, born into the Catholic faith and being Brazil's most respected medium, was eternally grateful to the "heroic" steps taken by the Catholic Church in bringing Christ to the lives of many in the New World. Chico, as he was best known, told the masses to be jubilant, that the pope had visited Brazil and along with the Catholic Church had contributed greatly to the many Christian-based faiths in Brazil.

Chico felt everyone should be grateful for the love sent forth by Christ to Brazil, through the Catholic Church. He also thanked his Creator for the freedom to think, discern, and follow any one of the many Christian based religions they chose. His eloquent, delicate, and Christ-like vocabulary would not tolerate anything other than respect and admiration for the Catholic Church.

This great spirit of light believed "To love God and all of His creation is to practice religion – the religion of God." Chico believed that a spiritual evolution that is illuminated by fraternal love, and goes hand in hand with the teachings of Christ, when practiced accordingly, would place humanity in a receptive mode to receive the immortal messages and teachings from superior beings of light. To understand

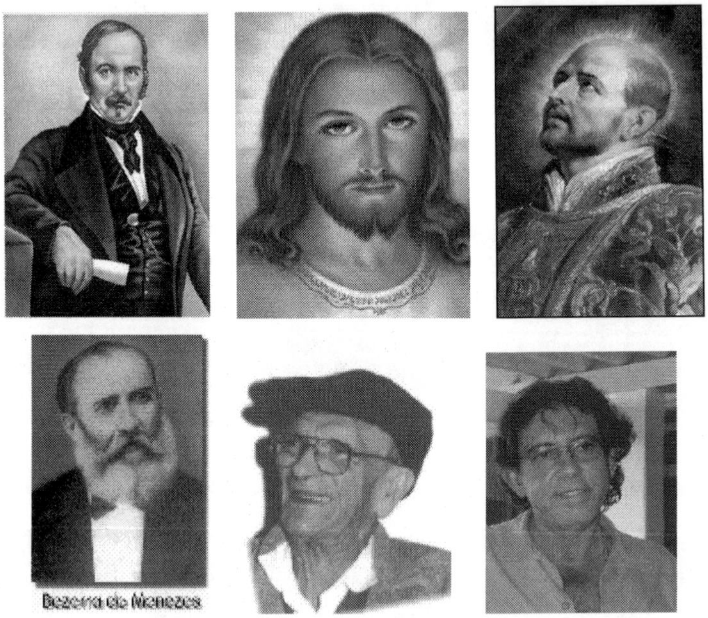

Clockwise, beginning with Jesus Christ at the top center, Saint Ignatius de Loyola, Healer João de Deus, Medium Chico Xavier, Dr. Adolfo Bezerra de Menezes, and the Father of Spiritism Allan Kardec.

these messages and assimilate all the lessons of progress they can minister to humanity, would bring order and progress to all.

Spending his life illuminating hearts, Chico Xavier, a messenger of peace, has been a pivotal figure in the history of Brazilian spirituality. Chico Xavier a pre-eminent world figure channeled more than four hundred books, following the illuminating messages of Kardec and Menezes. His books have been translated into dozens of languages. He gave all proceeds from his divine gift to the poor; never profited from any royalties.

Chico Xavier's most noteworthy achievement however, was his ability to reconcile the Kardecist-Spiritist Doctrine with traditional Catholicism, a monumental effort when considering the geographical size, multicultural diversity, and large Catholic population of Brazil (more than 2.5 million Spiritists, a majority who are also practicing Catholics), indicates many have identified with Chico Xavier's honest purpose.

By accomplishing such achievement, Chico Xavier creatively elaborated a new form of Brazilian popular Catholicism. Brazilians in order to transcend to Kardec's Christian-Spiritism had to replace long-established antagonistic systems characterized by traditional, institutional, and dogmatic order, with a more humane order of universal love, a genuine brotherhood.

A human embodiment of Christ-like consciousness, compassion, and humility, Chico Xavier is considered by many to be the Mother Theresa of Brazil. In 1981 he was nominated for the Nobel Peace Prize, and until his death in July 2002, he remained a most humble and loving expression of the teachings of Christ. Brazilians of all social classes loved him and continue to honor him to this date. Chico Xavier with his essential fraternal teachings of the Gospel of Christ has come to symbolize the prophesized "order and progress" imprinted on the Brazilian flag.

> *"To love God and all of His creation is to practice religion - the religion of God."*
> *- Chico Xavier*

The proverbial tolerance Brazilians have demonstrated (a result of the Catholic and Spiritist teachings) has also attracted a massive influx of Protestant denominations, starting at the end of the 19th century. These include Anglicans, Baptists, Lutherans, Methodists, and Presbyterians. After World War II new groups arrived, namely Jehovah Witnesses, Mormons, Pentecostals and adherents of the Four Square Gospel.

The Temple of Goodwill, in Brasilia, is perhaps Brazil's largest ecumenical center attracting dignitaries and spiritual leaders from all parts of the globe.

In São Paolo, the Archbishop of the Roman Catholic Church, Hummes, has gone on television speaking about the church. He is continuously trying to be more open to dialogue with science, reason, philosophy, culture, and society. He claims not to be a fundamentalist and sees important social, economic, and political issues as those that demand modern answers.

Brazil, in its immortal expression of spirit life, has come to represent for the entire world, the foundation of a new way of thinking. With the instrumental help of Kardec, Bezerra de Menezes, Chico Xavier, and healing phenomenon of Abadiania, João de Deus, as well as other genuine mediums, Brazil promises to be a country that will lead humanity to its greater self.

Professional classes have already organized themselves to study and extend the Doctrine paradigms in all professional areas, as can be seen in the National Congress of Spiritist Medical Doctors and the national (as well as international) organization of the Medical-Spiritist Association.

The Medical Spiritist Association whose mission is to contribute to the scientific studies and research of Medicine and Spiritism, aims to: educate health professionals about the importance of respecting and tolerating patient's beliefs and religions in practicing Spiritual Medicine; promote the medical-spiritist paradigm through courses and communication means, books and other publications; contribute with the implantation of this new medical paradigm throughout the world, and assist with the medical formation of creating more humanistic medical professionals and facilities.

2

SPIRIT HEALING WITHIN THE CONTEXT OF OTHER HEALING SYSTEMS AND BIOMEDICINE

Medical anthropology, the exciting field that looks at the way individuals throughout the world have approached issues of health, illness, and healing in their respective ways, has found that many ancient healing traditions still exist even though the civilizations that once practiced them have been non-existent for centuries. In the advent of a growing popularity for alternative or complementary methods of healing, many of these old traditions are making a comeback. In comparing modern medicine to ancient methods of healing, some similarities are found, with the most significant difference being the missing spiritual element from the current biomedical model.

The classification of diseases of supernatural etiology has been completely disregarded by classic medicine. It is important to keep in mind that the exclusion of a spiritual classification of disease in the current classic model, does not mean it does not exist, it simply means the medical establishment chose not to include it in the current classification. We need only to recall cosmology (the science that deals with the systematic origin and structure of the universe) in its earlier years of development, was based solely on metaphysical examination. Eventually, after much efficient and rigorous study, cosmology did gain acceptance to the physical sciences. It is only a matter of time before spiritual/psychic healing becomes an accepted field in classic scientific medicine.

The wealth of medical knowledge that is available to us from many of the ancient world healing systems validates important cosmological and theological principles that are missing from today's modern medicine. Common among these ancient traditions are: 1) the importance of a harmonious balance (inner and external) in achieving health, 2) working with the human energy fields, 3) modification of lifestyle, diet, and exercise, 4) *the existence of spirits in disease and the supernatural dimension of healing (faith and prayer),* 5) and the ideologies of true knowledge, purity, harmony, and goodness. Important aspects of health are prevention (through diet, exercise, relaxation/meditation/ritual), detoxification, and regulating the humors to achieve physical, emotional, and mental balance.

Interestingly the Japanese concept of purification: keeping the rules of life correctly, according to the laws of nature, should equally provide optimal health and quality of life. Purification emphasizes cleanliness of both the internal and external bodies. Considering Japanese people today, have the highest longevity rates, it is definitely worth consideration.

"In comparing modern medicine to ancient methods of healing, some similarities are found, with the most significant difference being the missing spiritual element from the current biomedical model."

Another important feature of eastern medicine, particularly Tibetan/Buddhist medicine, is that they explicitly name *compassion* as the most fundamental aspect of medicine. Each of the eastern healing traditions represents a complete system of medicine, and each takes into account the patient's environment, diet, behavior, mental state, and also the seasons, celestial cycles, and spirit influence.

From the western world - Mesoamerican and Native American traditions - we find natives have included anatomy, diagnostics, therapeutics, and theories of cosmology and theology into their medical repertoire. Native American and Mesoamerican groups had a codified system of medicine before the first medical school was built in the new world, meaning that before the arrival of the Europeans, indigenous peoples were by no means primitive.

At the root of all these ancient healing traditions is the ultimate goal of the spirit liberating itself. We find the same element in Brazilian spiritual healing. With all due respect, the spiritual life Portuguese Latin Americans have come to know surpasses the religious sense. Brazilians compared to their Spanish Latin American counterparts have taken on a stronger "spiritual" (vs. religious) character. While mediumistic healing has definitely had a place in Spanish Latin American culture and healing traditions, it has existed covertly behind the larger traditional dogmatic ideology of institutionalized religion, which in Spanish Latin America has been predominantly represented by the Catholic Church.

Spanish Latin America, being more "dogmatic" in its religious character, does not permit it's members to participate in or believe in the reality of *curanderismo* (folk healing), particularly, mediumistic healing practices. Any attempt to make contact with disincarnate spirits is entirely prohibited. They are however permitted to pray in fellowship with angels and canonized saints. And while the concept of reincarnation has never been part of the dogma taught by the church, it has been the topic of growing discussion among biblical scholars critically analyzing missing and edited Christian Gospels.

While it could only be speculation at this point, perhaps omitting the subject of reincarnation from church teachings will soon come to be explained as an issue that served the political and military interests of the times. Whether or not reincarnation is, or is not a reality, is not the main point here. What is relevant and should be a central point is the importance of living the present life in harmony and in brotherhood, by living life with the love, truth, justice, and peace of the Creator.

For Brazilians Spiritists it is only a matter of time before the truth is revealed about the current secular world. They understand that changing and manipulating the truths of the universe, the natural forces of nature have been antagonized, reflecting on the entire social, economic, and political order.

Living in a secular world that is primarily focused on the acquisition of things, and often too many times, characterized by selfishness, has caused humanity to not only lose many valuable aspects of the human experience, but has also had to disguise them with other truths. This is a serious problem, particularly as these common misconceptions affect all aspects of human life. This has been the case for Dr. Stanley Krippner. Note the following observation he made during an interview with Jeffrey Mishlove, PhD., regarding spiritual healing as a phenomenon that tends to be disguised with a mystical cult or sorcery:

"You know the worst black magic is the black magic we commit against ourselves. It is the sorcery that hurts ourselves when we think negative thoughts, or we hold onto a destructive self-concept, or when we allow ourself to say negative, hostile things about ourselves and the people around us, and those sentences go over and over in our mind. It is no wonder, then, that people get stomach aches and backaches and headaches with those negative thought images going around. And yes, to me that sounds like something that's sorcery, and that can be exorcised, so much the better. If you want to call this a malevolent spirit fine. If you want to call it negative thinking fine. But either the spiritist or the psychotherapist, or both of them, really have to approach that negativity and get rid of it if the person's going to recover" (Mishlove, 1998).

Undeniably, grasping the sacredness of spirit healing (with the assistance of benevolent spirits), cannot be experienced equally by all, particularly if the sacredness of life is not equally perceived by everyone. Discernment, the spirit of truth takes on new meaning here.

An example is demonstrated in the Christian Gospel when Jesus speaks to people at the temple about his messiahship. "You cannot hear the voice of God, because your ears are closed. You cannot comprehend the works of God, because your hearts are full of self. And you are busybodies, mischief-makers, hypocrites. You take these men whom God has given me into your haunts and try to poison them with sophistries and lies, and think that you will snatch them from the fold of God" (Dowling, 1979, p. 214, line

8). Some people attempt to stone Jesus, but he stops them and asks them for which of his good works is He being stoned for? Healing the sick, or expelling evil spirits?

Through modernization, secularization, and technological advances the spirit of truth has undeniably been distorted, directly affecting all value systems and the sacredness of life, as is illustrated by a major political failure to provide adequate healthcare services to everyone alike, particularly when this occurs in industrialized nations as the case with the United States.

From a technicist standpoint, most conventional medical schools have taught illness as a series of technical problems that are to be approached with an application of specific technical solutions. A value system that is then reinforced in practice by the expectations of the public and by the requirements of the regulators and governing agencies has consequently given greater value to technical excellence. As a result society has professional medical performance that is excellent in technical terms but poor in humanistic terms as can be observed in our healthcare system's evolutionary path.

This has generated a host of adverse ill effects on health outcomes. Serving different populations in different ways (primarily distinguished by socio-economic class) the American Healthcare system fails to distribute its resources equally among its entire patient population. Even within the subsystem that serves the poor in this country there is great reluctance to treat disadvantaged patient groups. Many health practitioners choose not to become Medi-Caid (Medi-Cal) providers, and decline treatment to these underserved patients simply because of the negative impact, low reimbursements will have on their medical practice's financial viability.

While the economic and political arguments are of extreme importance in understanding the inequities of the healthcare system, they are beyond the scope of this particular work. The sacredness of the medical vocation however is important here. How both, folk medicine and biomedicine differ from this essential "sacred" reference point should be significant in understanding why the two, work and produce, strikingly different outcomes.

Underlining the difference between conventional medicine and folk medicine traditions, Finkler notes "Spiritualism is embedded in a sacred world while biomedicine is sanctioned by secular science" (1994, p. 179). According to Finkler, folk medicine, and biomedical models have different physical settings, etiological beliefs, diagnosis and treatment repertoire, reasons for practicing, the difference in the practitioner-patient relationship, as it relates to their particular focus.

Ms. Finkler contends that in biomedicine the focus of a patient's healing is on the physician, his persona, knowledge, and reputation. The patient who followed the doctor's treatment plan, and got desired results, or even an undesired outcome, attributes the results to the physician. He got better (or worse) because of the doctor's ability (or inability) to cure him. In this model the patient looks to the doctor for the alleviation of his/her suffering. The patient even after diet modification, and following the doctor's plan of treatment rigidly, waits for the healing to occur. Here the doctor only treats the effect of the disease.

> *"The patient who followed the doctor's treatment plan, and got desired results, or even an undesired outcome, attributes the results to the physician. He got better (or worse) because of the doctor's ability (or inability) to cure him. In this model the patient looks to the doctor for the alleviation of his/her suffering." - Finkler*

In contrast, the focus of folk/spiritual healing is on the patient. In this case the healer (many times guided by spirit entities) removes the "evil spirits" that are causing the disease. The patient may receive relief from his ill symptoms, mostly attributed to the spiritual cleansing and purification practices conducted by folk healers and their spirit assistants. Brazilian spiritual healing, like Mexican spiritual healing described by Finkler, emphasizes self-responsibility in their individual care, and health outcomes. Their different focus,' is therefore the fundamental difference between spiritual healing and biomedicine. Classic medicine, ruled by technicism and by a reductionist-materialistic character, has come to exacerbate the doctor-patient relationship.

As if it had drawn from the ancient healing traditions of the east, and the original inhabitants of Africa and America, Brazil has been one of the few nations in the world to synthesize this vast and invaluable medical, philosophical, and spiritual (moral) knowledge from some of the world's greatest healing and spiritual traditions, and efficiently construct a most useful and effective model of integral health.

Although similar to the spiritual component found in universal holistic and homeopathic health models, Brazil's spiritual concept differs slightly, specifically its use of mediumistic healing techniques. Working with the help of benevolent spirits may initially sound bizarre and almost impossible for many to conceptualize and not until one becomes better informed and discerned by way of independent study, can one make a sound assessment. Having said this, I propose the reader see Brazilian spiritual healing not from his particular worldview but rather from the unique Brazilian mindset.

A Spiritual Healing Model of Health Overview

For Brazilians, achieving integral health requires the soul be in a pure state of existence, or at least for it to be in a constant purification process. This is accomplished through individual efforts of work, study (specifically spiritual education, educating the soul), and activities of good works. Educating the soul with fundamental moral concepts of the laws of nature is what Brazilians believe create the personal transformation that is required for complete healing.

Much of this spiritual knowledge is gained through knowledge of the Christian Gospel, and an extension of it, the Spiritist Doctrine (*Kardecismo)* – a scientific, philosophical, and moral way of life that promotes preventative care and a more complete diagnostic and treatment regimen for many known and unknown medical conditions.

Unlike the classic model of medicine, the relationship between soul and body is inextricably linked to a person's health. Without adequate diagnosis (many having origins in the soul) and inappropriate treatment, higher levels of consciousness cannot be achieved, personal transformation is inevitably hindered, and healing, may not take true effect.

The Christian Spiritist doctrine which highlights cosmic principles of reincarnation, karma, the law of cause and effect, as well as fraternal charity – are believed to contribute to a greater understanding of the meaning and purpose of individual life within the greater context of humanity's evolution.

From a health perspective the doctrine provides a clear and ample connection between a person's moral condition (the soul's condition), the balance or imbalance of their energetic organism, and their current health condition (in other words, a strong interrelationship between soul, *perispirit*, and body respectively). Thus, Brazilians who live by the doctrine, find the concepts of health and illness to be more profoundly defined than the limited definitions known by the current conventional medical paradigm.

A central tenet of spiritual healing is that everything, including health and illness, occurs around the Theory of Relativity found in quantum physics and the spiritual Law of Reciprocity. When the *soul* is in equilibrium with the *perispirit* (the semi-material, spiritual and physical, human envelope) and *physical body*, the individual enjoys good health, but when disequilibrium occurs, disease sets in.

For healing to occur, love must become the predominant energy. Ideals of transformation (such as changing lifestyle, diet modifications, personal changes toward a better self, one that will also improve all relationships) must be applied in order that a person's vital energetic centers are reactivated. Consequently, it should restore the patient's spiritual purpose and cosmic equilibrium that should harmonize any imbalance found in the individual, and could ultimately restore the patient's ill-health.

3

THE SCIENTIFIC, PHILOSOPHICAL, AND MORAL ASPECTS OF BRAZILIAN MEDICINE

Brazilian doctors trained in modern medicine who practice the Spiritist way of life as well as other non-Brazilian physicians who are rediscovering a renewed sense of sacredness in scientific medicine now acknowledge the great need to study beyond the physical-chemical phenomena related to the person's biological metabolism. They believe classic medicine has reduced studies to only the organic body and has completely ignored the multi-dimensional aspect of the human organism.

The current allopathic psychiatric model, too, follows a purely organic etiology in mental functioning as it has been structured within the complexities of the neuro-endocrine metabolism. The soul as it relates to healing, under a purely scientific standpoint has been most commonly rejected, claiming to exist only outside the empirical arena, and not fitting into the standard observation, measurement and experimentation of research investigation.

The soul lacking the attention it deserves, is short of a scientific explanation. This has made the soul non-verifiable, non-existent, and therefore difficult to explain or comprehend in scientific terms. However, for Brazilians who believe it is their natural legacy to develop this area of scientific inquiry, spiritual healing is not about presenting information that has no basis or validity. The public is not expected to accept information crudely. Rather, spiritual healing in Brazil is a legitimate field of inquiry that has been and continues to be approached critically at the scientific, philosophical, and moral level.

If everything that is scientifically analyzed provides a rational interpretation, then spiritual healing is scientific. We know most physiological and biological processes are based on chemical interactions, which can be accounted for. Simply put, the general subject matter of all sciences is the inter-behavior of two or more phenomenon (in biology the inter-behavior of organisms with their environment, and in psychology the inter-behavior of organisms with other organisms or with inorganic objects).

The behavior between organisms (whether organic and/or inorganic) together under the conditions with which they interact, constitute fields with definite boundaries. In the case of spiritual/psychic healing, the basic principle behind this healing modality has been established, not by spiritual healers, but by scientific research of material things. Science has demonstrated beyond a shadow of a doubt, that nothing ever takes place without a cause and each cause results in some form of effect.

Unlike what many people think, spiritual healing is not explained by myth, but rather by validating disciplines of science, medicine, biology, physiology, medical anthropology, cosmology, theology, philosophy, religion, parapsychology, theistic psychology, and quantum physics.

Increasing scientific discoveries, in particular discoveries related to transpersonal psychology, have recently opened new horizons for the study and interpretation of many psychic phenomenon, recognizing established concepts of consciousness, sub-consciousness, and superconsciousness. Growing interest and study of the faculty of mediumship, in particular *healing mediumship* (psychic healing), now permits us to classify it scientifically as a psychobiological predisposition inherent to those who under certain conditions are allowed to capture the thoughts of disincarnate spirits, can experience the astral plane, and can also establish contact with the spirit world. Brazilians, studying the organic and psychic phenomena of mediumship for more than a century, are leading the world in establishing essential understanding of mediumistic healing principles.

Modern day investigations of spiritual healing demonstrate healers possess energetic fields with unique properties that allow an actual exchange of energy between healer and patient. Researchers such as Sister Justa Smith, a biochemist, have found spiritual healing not to be the result of psychosomatic effects, as has been a common misconception for centuries. Dr. Smith's research suggests that healers have the ability to selectively affect different enzyme systems in a direction toward greater organization and energy balance (Smith, 1973).

By speeding up different enzymatic reactions, healers assist the body in healing itself; something allopathic physicians are not trained to do. Healers therefore provide the patient with the needed energetic boost to push the patient's total energetic system back into homeostasis. A healing boost of this magnitude has special negatively entropic, self-organizational properties that assist the cells in creating order from disorder along selectively defined routes of cellular expression. This, as well as other, recent discoveries involving plants and animals are scientific examples of a healer's effect on the healing process of biological organisms.

"By speeding up different enzymatic reactions, healers assist the body in healing itself; something allopathic physicians are not trained to do."

It is important to note that the biological organisms that are mentioned in this study were all non-human. The animal (mice), plant, and enzyme systems were utilized instead of a human being to remove the suggestion or belief on the part of the test subject. Such studies demonstrate the validity of the existence of a concretely observed and measured therapeutic energy exchange between healers and biological systems.

These research studies direct us to further investigate the energetic body. The future of medical advances may well be in our ability to control such energy, and in helping people in ways we have not, as yet, been able to do. It is research studies such as these that have left some scientists with a firm conviction that magnetic fields play an important role in the body's healing and immunological processes.

The field of parapsychology has been supported with the works contributed by Professor Michael Persinger, head of the Neuroscience Research Group (Psychophysiology Laboratory) at Laurentian University in Canada. His hypotheses that the extremely low frequency (ELF) Shumann waves may serve as carrier for *psi* information (psychic phenomena involving the sixth sense, i.e. channeling, clairsentience, clairvoyance, clairaudience, automatic writing, distant healing, mental telepathy, etc.) resulted positive. Most interesting however, is his observation of the variation in the earth's geomagnetic field. The area having the lowest magnetic intensity on the planet is in Brazil, near Rio de Janeiro. This geographical advantage in terms of the growing psychic phenomenon and spirituality in Brazil, could explain their ability to communicate with the spirit world and to potentially lead the world in its spiritual evolution.

While scientific research on the health benefits of prayer is still in it's infancy, and while some of the studies done on the effect of prayer on the therapeutic process have shown it has no effect on the therapeutic process there is still a small and growing body of evidence of the positive effect prayer has on overall health and well being. In the *Handbook of Religion and Health* (2001), Koenig, McCullough and Larson acknowledge intercessory prayer to be good for one's health (both mental and physical health). In their review of 1200 research studies and 400, reviews, they found religious involvement to be a direct correlation with many aspects of healthy living (e.g. well-being, happiness, fulfillment, greater hope and optimism, less anxiety and greater purpose and meaning of life).

In yet another source supporting these findings, *The Relaxation Response* (2000), Dr. Herbert Benson a Harvard behavioral medicine specialist has studied the effect of meditation and prayer on health for over thirty years. In his book he shows that patients can successfully overcome many stress related ailments by repeating a word, a sound, or a prayer. At his Institute for mind/body medicine, his effective and essential self-care modalities are growing in acceptance to potentially become a third modality in health care, next to surgical interventions and pharmaceuticals.

Also regarding the positive effect spirituality has on the therapeutic process are the findings from Larson, Milano, and Lu (1988), researchers who also investigated the effect of prayer on healing. They have found it is a research area that has definite benefits for humanity and thus requires further investigation. Despite the published studies, which have demonstrated religion's ameliorating effect on patient's suffering, and lowering self-destructive behaviors to aid in the promotion of a healthy lifestyle, the empirical evidence has not received the proper attention nor have they received the appropriate research focus.

Undoubtedly, research findings continue to support the claim that it is those patients whom lack spirituality who are at greater risk for illness. Additional support for these claims has also been offered by Dr. Dale Matthews of Georgetown University. Matthews has found 75% of the studies performed on the effect spirituality has on the healing process, are beneficial. The need for a spiritual dimension provides meaning to life. This has definite physiological consequences.

As Dr. Raphi Kelman points out, "If we can't get patients to activate their interest in meaning (however they define it) we will not be successful in healing" (Lerner, 2000, p. 215). Kelman, as well as Rabbi Michael Lerner's message, point to society's collective denial of the spirit and how this has systematically repressed our human needs, specifically how this has repressed our perception of health and illness. It is the dualistic philosophical theory of spirit and matter, health and illness, good and evil, natural and supernatural, that Brazilians believe offers humanity a better understanding of medicine.

Only when the two realms of science and religion come to terms with one another, will this be achieved. The great *philosophical* significance in spiritual healing offers solid and logical answers to humanity's eternal questions.... *where do we come from? ..... where are we going*?

> *"The need for a spiritual dimension in our lives provides meaning to life. This has definite physiological consequences."*

Unlike classic medicine, spiritual healing reestablishes the connection between the patient and the greater cosmic principles of his/her existence, those of karma (cause and effect), and reincarnation, which in the treatment protocols help identify a true etiology for a patient's ailment. Spiritual healing offers above all, philosophical depth, promoting a revolution of ideas and critical thinking about the individual and it's world, particularly where social, political, economic, health, and moral conditions are irrational.

Since the exploration of emotions, feelings, thoughts and ideas, cannot be expressed in material or physical terms alone [because human consciousness (the soul), requires it be studied from the less explored, spiritual realm of knowledge], a broader understanding will occur when investigators reach beyond the human (physical) senses. Such transcendental knowledge that goes beyond the realm of sense is found in the teachings of Christ. In the *Aquarian Gospel*, Jesus enlightens Greek philosophers of the seen and unseen realities:

"I come not here to speak of science, of philosophy, or art: of these you are the world's best masters now. But all your high accomplishments are but stepping-stones to worlds beyond the realm of sense; are but illusive shadows flitting on the walls of time. But I will tell you of a life beyond, within; a real life that cannot pass away. ... Unaided by the Spirit-breath, the work of intellection tends to solve the problems of the things we see, and nothing more. The senses were ordained to bring into the mind mere pictures of the things that pass away; they do not deal with real things; they do not comprehend eternal law. But man has something in his soul a something that will tear the veil apart that he may see the world of real things. We call this something, spirit consciousness; it sleeps in every soul, and cannot be awakened till the Holy Breath becomes a welcome guest .... There is no power in intellect to turn the key; philosophy and science both have toiled to get a glimpse behind the veil; but they have failed. The secret spring that throws ajar the door of soul is touched by nothing else than purity in life, by prayer and holy thought" (Dowling, 1979, p. 84).

An insightful message, that neither science nor philosophy *alone* have all the answers and will gain the ability to find true meaning in everything only when they both develop a keen sense of discrimination and discernment, through a greater moral understanding.

Man through his inborn powers and knowledge of the kingdom of the soul is naturally led to his higher self. *Genuine* healers (mediumistic and psychic) possess advanced understanding of the spirit realm. Only through individual evolutionary effort is discernment gained, a critical extra-sensorial perception that is dormant until awakened in the human soul.

Lastly, spiritual healing as Brazilians know it, requires a *moral* understanding of essential human aptitudes: universal love, a sense of justice, respect, and tolerance of others (fraternal solidarity), as these are essential natural instruments that allow the individual to live in perfect harmony with his surroundings, and thus allows him to live his physical existence in a more complete and balanced way.

"Spiritual healing offers above all, philosophical depth, promoting a revolution of ideas and critical thinking about the individual and it's world, particularly where social, political, economic, health, and moral conditions are irrational."

A greater moral understanding, achieved through educating the soul with divinely inspired lessons (Christian as well as other enlightening spiritual teachings that come from many other world spiritual traditions), will help individuals better acquaint themselves with the ideology of good and aid the patient in finding genuine purpose.

Major ideals of personal transformation require one love everyone (especially, those poor in spirit, and one's enemies), and one constantly be involved in working for the *common* good. A true worker for the collective progress of humanity shows compassion and forgiveness, applies faith to all aspects of everyday life, practices fraternal charity and humility, and conscientiously uses and distributes personal wealth by detaching from worldly possessions.

Through love (the catalyst of morality), a person who dedicates himself to the service and lives of others reinvigorates his life depending on the tone and degree of benevolent acts he accomplishes. It is important for love and knowledge to continue to work together, as knowledge without love can result in self-destruction or insanity, and love without knowledge can lead to fanaticism.

Man has more easily succumbed to the shadow of dogma, orthodoxy, politics, and greed – all distant forces from the center of God's creation. Distancing oneself from God hinders a true understanding of consciousness. Without a genuine understanding of what a conscious life demands from all mortals [reverence to nature (God), and cooperation among all humans] achieving Oneness, or Unity (the perfect balance and equilibrium), becomes an almost impossible task. Thus if it is non-centeredness that has caused humanity to become ill, an effective plan of treatment should be one that allows one to realign with the central point one has drifted from.

"Man through his inborn powers and knowledge of the kingdom of the soul is naturally led to his higher self."

Faith, optimism, and prayer, experienced in a climate of hope along with the help and guidance of the Spirit-breath are the most valuable resources humans have in the possibility of regaining health. Moral flab and laziness will finally be overcome when humanity has grown exponentially in consciousness, to the point where there is no difference between individual will and that of Divine will.

PART TWO

MAXIMIZING SPIRIT MEDICINE

4

CONCEPTS OF THE BRAZILIAN SPIRITUAL WORLDVIEW

The purpose of this section is to introduce three significant elements that constitute Brazilian spiritual healing: *the human soul and it's relationship to immortality, the human energy system, and the role of human emotions in health and illness*. Perhaps when these three are better understood by the biomedical world, the ill symptoms of a patient can be better understood, more completely diagnosed, more efficiently and effectively treated, in terms of final health outcomes, and in terms of cost-effectiveness.

The Human Soul

For Brazilians the soul and spirit are in fact two aspects of a single entity. In other words the soul/spirit is a continuum of a sacred unity that connects the vibrational aspect of the spiritual being, to the material aspect of the human being. The soul is that which lives in the biological body and participates in the constitution of the human body. As soul, the spirit takes on a biologically evolutionary form in order to purify and become more lucid through the earthly knowledge and experiences it acquires. All souls are created *equal*, simple and ignorant.

"According to the Spiritist doctrine there are not many lives, but rather one eternal life with various phases of evolution, in different physical incarnations."

Through successive rebirths in different physical bodies (reincarnation) the soul acquires through it's own effort and free will, conditions that allow for higher levels of consciousness. Reincarnation in accordance with the Law of Immortality of the Soul, contends the soul survives physical death and makes available the opportunity to participate in a new existence (a new biological form), in order that it may reach its highest level of evolution, and maintain its individuality throughout the successive incarnations.

Reincarnation allows a faulty soul from a previous incarnation the opportunity to be born again to correct previous errors, negligence or indifferences. For spirits who have no errors to correct, reincarnation allows the soul to gain the greatest level of spiritual evolution. According to the Spiritist doctrine there are *not* many lives, but rather *one* eternal life with various phases of evolution, in different physical incarnations.

The reincarnated soul is not a newborn to this planet, as it brings with it a predisposition directly related to it's previous lives – influences, knowledge, and experiences that remain imprinted in the soul. This fundamental concept of reincarnation, a central pillar of Spiritism, is intricately related to the concepts of human imperfection, disease, and suffering. Disease, in the context of human suffering is seen as the purifying agent, necessary for the soul to evolve.

After physical death, this entity is no longer "soul" and instead is transformed to "spirit" outside the physical body, as it now exists free in the spirit realm. It is at this point that the spirit entity is no longer considered part of living physical matter. The soul when not united with a body is a spirit.

"A spirit is not an abstract, undefined being, only to be conceived of by our thought; it is a real, circumscribed being which in certain cases, is appreciated by the senses of sight, hearing, and touch. Spirits belong to different order; they are not equals either in power, intelligence, knowledge, or moral excellence. Those in the highest order are distinguished by purity, knowledge, and love of goodness – they are often called "angels" or "pure spirits." The others are relatively more distant from this perfection. Those in the lower orders are inclined to most of our human passions (hate, envy, jealousy, pride, etc.) and may still take pleasure in wrong-doing" (Kardec, 2003, p. 11).

It is spirit entities from the higher order who no longer need to reincarnate to the physical plane that assist mediumistic healers. These spirits continue to elevate in the spirit plane by the extent of their benevolence.

It is the natural Law of Cause and Effect that becomes manifest in this or future phases of the evolutionary path. According to this rigorous law, each person receives according to what deeds he has practiced (good, bad, productive or unproductive, etc.), particularly as practiced for the common good. This natural law is the culmination of the lesson in Christ's Parable of the Sower, teaching one reaps what one has sowed.

"The reincarnated soul is not a newborn to this planet, as it brings with it predispositions directly related to it's previous lives – influences, knowledge, and experiences that remain imprinted in the soul."

A modality of the Law of Cause and Effect, Karmic Law, is related to grave errors in one's evolutionary biography. Health conditions deriving from karmic causes manifest from birth (e.g. congenital conditions, and birth defects) or during the course of the person's present life. Karma often appears without apparent cause or without a physical or medical explanation and may be attributed to faults committed by the soul in the past. Considered cosmic law manifesting itself in the physical plane, karma's finality is to bring harmony by way of encouraging a review of one's belief system and doing all one can do to bring it into harmony with the Laws of the universe.

Karmic Law thus becomes the natural "equalizer" that allows individuals to see their hardships, difficulties, and suffering as past actions or inactions they must now tend to or repair, in order to harmonize the cosmic imbalance it originally created. Expiation, and reparation are the best therapeutic modalities, and are necessary in eliminating the spiritual, psychological, emotional, and physical ill effects brought about by past errors.

Alone, forgiveness coming from Divine grace is necessary in order to delete human error, but individual expiation and reparation are also necessary to restore individual, societal, and cosmic balance. Understanding that a great deal of infractions (individual and collective) are committed in the presence of laws that regulate human behavior, has helped patients understand their suffering as the result of their own free-will.

Forgiving therefore involves genuine compassion, that releases the offense and the debtor, and that transforms the individual's ill health to greater moral and social health. For Brazilians this is not difficult to do, as they know this is the key to the Principle of the Universal Paternity, it is what unlocks the brotherhood. Their concept of "today one of us, tomorrow another one of us" enables Brazilians to help those seeking a fraternal solicitation, in giving them a helping hand, or more importantly, a gentle and edifying word, or gesture. Brazilians see it as everyone's equal obligation to aid those brothers and sisters who are in need, are weak, ignorant, and morally inferior, to be helped to their greater self.

By learning to cultivate selflessness, Brazilians are teaching their brothers to become active members of the social and moral renovation of the planet. Brazilians not only believe compassion, and charitable fraternal works are essential, they also insist on justly preserving them, continuously fermenting them, and constructing them as something that is indispensable for all humanity.

Building a spirit of renewal, particularly by sharing the Word with those in need of spiritual and moral values contained in the Gospel, Brazilians are generating greater understanding of the importance of renouncing to transitory things as the only way to getting more energetically involved in the progress of humanity.

Solidarity, the constructor of all edifying ideals, of unselfish servants working to construct an ideal brotherhood, has gained new meaning in Brazilian society. Societal life, the balance of opposing and contrary forces, is ideally described as a perfect state when order, peace, and harmony exist among all peoples. When one of these is out of synchrony with the other it creates much discord, confusion, and needless suffering.

This is why Brazilians are working to instill in the hearts and minds of all people a profound awareness of the consequences of thoughts and deeds that are brought to humanity. The intervention of the invisible world, they find, is necessary to awaken “indifferent” souls to the notion of immortality and to the cosmic obligation the heavens demand of all mortal beings.

The solidarity that Brazilians exemplify goes beyond the basics of the principles of solidarity as is most commonly known. We see the fraternal assistance provided at the core of all spiritist centers as one that is done genuinely to assist brothers and sisters in need.

This concept of Brazilian solidarity is intricately connected to the afterlife and is best described through the process of charity. A charity that is not limited to caring for the immediate corporal, physiological, and emotional needs of the physically needy, but rather is one that contains a deeper sense and involves the intended liberation of conscience. A freedom that is achieved through freeing the being of it’s own ignorance, of what is keeping the soul from spiritually ascending. The realization of Spirit is helping humans renounce to self to be better able to ease the pain and suffering of others, of lifting others to a healthier, happier, and higher state. This is the sign of a new evolution for our times.

As it is noted in The Supreme Mystery: “All of those who are in a condition of unhappiness in the world are that way because of desiring their own release. All of those who are in a condition of happiness in the world are that way from seeking the release of another.” Making energetic progress toward the common good is part of the doctrine of Infinite

Growth as taught by Chico Xavier. Teaching to co-fraternize with others, particularly sharing the Word with respect to spiritual and moral values, to assist those brothers and sisters who are living in darkness, in discord, in bitterness, and in selfishness, is making energetic progress toward the common good. Chico Xavier understood that individual progress and more importantly, collective progress, are defined by the condition of the soul or souls that create it.

> *"Considered cosmic law manifesting itself in the physical plane, karma's finality is to bring harmony by way of encouraging a review of one's belief system and doing all one can do to bring it into harmony with the Laws of the universe."*

As difficulties and challenges surmount, working and serving others and forgetting oneself in the midst of it all becomes the best answer. As Chico Xavier recommended to his following: "Work more, by serving more." The same message with exact meaning is found in the Gospel teachings of Christ, instructing humanity not to work for the food that does not last, but rather to work for the food that gives eternal life.

Charity as practiced by Brazilian spiritists is not one that gives from material excesses, nor is it one that gives from the things no longer needed or no longer wanted but rather is one that gives from what is treasured most, the heart; giving with a sincere disposition to serve.

By helping others unfold themselves in their superior purpose it is clear that God has left humanity the work to complete each other, to complete the earth, to complete God's creation, thus making humans completely responsible for the outcome of their planetary existence. Understanding that everyone is part of the whole - part of the eternal order of all things

– redefines human values, our human obligation to this planet and to all beings.

Appreciating the value of the interconnection of all life and equally partaking in the transformation of reality through the service of others, Brazilians are showing the world that everyone is indispensable in the making of the planet, in the making of their own life, and their own health. Creating a fearless, peaceful, and selfless planet is only a genuine "care" away.

"The intervention of the invisible world, they find, is necessary to awaken "indifferent" souls to the notion of immortality and to the cosmic obligation the heavens demand of all mortal beings."

Now before bringing this section to an end, it is important to clarify two important terms that tend to be used interchangeably in Brazilian spiritual healing, *spiritualist and spiritist* require some clarification. A spiritualist refers to someone who adheres to the philosophy that human beings are more than just matter. All religions that accept the existence of a principle independent from matter, in the human being, are spiritualist. However in the American and British usage, it is more clearly defined as a belief that the dead communicate with the living through mediums. While there are many parallels between spiritualism and the spiritist doctrine, the differences are very significant and should not be confused, or used as equivalents.

A spiritist as defined by Allan Kardec refers to someone who adheres to the philosophy that deals with the origin, nature, and destiny of spirits as well as their relationship with the corporeal world. As a science, Spiritism can be seen as the search of the truth of humanity's spiritual nature with the principle objective of helping humanity heal, progress, and evolve. Spiritists believe their practice is not one that communicates with the dead. Rather, they believe their mediums communicate with the Spirit of Truth – communicating concepts of truth that can offer lasting freedom to humanity.

While both spiritists and spiritualists observe eternal progress as a central tenet of their philosophy, all spiritists believe in the central teaching of reincarnation, in achieving this progress; whereas not all spiritualists necessarily accept the concept of reincarnation. Clearly both spiritualist and spiritist believe in a life that goes beyond physical matter but only the latter believes in utilizing the valuable knowledge, resources and assistance (goes beyond the sensorial aspect to spirit incorporation) from the Spirit realm with the only objective of helping humanity heal, progress, and evolve.

5

THE RELATIONSHIP BETWEEN SOUL, MIND, BODY, HEALTH AND ILLNESS

It is within a comprehensive understanding of the soul and perispirit that mediumistic healers diagnose physical disease. Diagnosing illness within the spiritual paradigm, requires healing mediums understand that many health problems patients have, spring from emotional, mental, and spiritual imbalances; for healing to occur, *all* of these imbalances must first be identified, adequately addressed, carefully and individually treated. "Medicine considering only the material (physical) aspect, is deprived of an incessant cause of action. Knowledge of the *peri-spirit* is the key to a crowd of medical problems hitherto inexplicable" (Estrich-Pellegrino, 1997, p. 79).

The perispirit (formed of subtle wrappings of atoms) is the semi-material envelope that links the soul and the body during biological life; it is the means by which the soul (spirit) acts upon matter, and matter acts upon soul (spirit). Spiritual influence has biological repercussion, and psycho-organic behaviors have influence upon spirit. The mind, in housing feelings and emotions, turns out to be a more powerful agent in generating disease and disharmony, than are known bacteria and viruses. The physical body, within the spiritual paradigm, therefore serves as the impurity filter of the soul and provides the means for it's spiritual evolution.

As spiritual beings living a physical experience (unlike physical beings having a spiritual experience), there is a reciprocal force between soul and body, a merging of responsibility that takes place in the human mind. The soul being an important constituent of the human being is the center of all it's potentiality, where all human thoughts begin to take form. It stores character, determination, thoughts, intelligence, will, ethics, intuition, conscience, personal artistic talents, scientific literacy, and religious perception.

According to Dr. Roberto Brolio the differences in human behaviors are fundamentally related to the soul, since their thought, intellect, will, free-choice, as well as other psychic manifestations which characterize the way the person thinks and acts, are shaped by the soul's predisposition.

The soul's attributes characterize human individuality and were not imposed by God, but by the individual's free will and efforts of work, study and other endeavors, in this as well as other incarnations. Since the soul is immortal, it does not age, it evolves by acquiring knowledge and experiences, enhancing it's individuality throughout time. This explains a small child who presents itself with a higher intellect than most children of the same age; sometimes displaying more intellectual abilities and spiritual aspiration than some adults whom never show any signs of enlightenment and who have gone through their physical existence with a mediocre rate of spiritual growth.

The soul (conscience) containing the totality of knowledge acquired throughout its entire existence, contains organic, psychic and spiritual aspects of the human being, which is formed by the conscience, sub-conscience, and super-conscience. These three areas of the human brain (rooms of the mental house), balance and restore the forces of the physical organism.

> *"The soul being an important constituent of the human being is the center of all it's potentiality, where all human thoughts begin to take form. It stores character, determination, thoughts, intelligence, will, ethics, intuition, conscience, personal artistic talents, scientific literacy, and religious perception."*

Brazilian healthcare professionals understanding how thought comes before form (emotional, physiological and/or biological forms), and consciousness exists before matter, can approach all morbid processes as essentially being mentally-commanded by the soul. Suely Caldas Schubert, Brazilian Spiritist-psychologist in her book *Os Poderes da Mente* (*The Powers of the Mind*) (2004) emphasizes the mind's capabilities as being totally dependent on the soul. The soul's attributes produce a chain of thoughts that are sorted and directed in the mental house which is composed of (1) the primary brain, (2) cortex motor, and (3) frontal lobes.

The primary brain (our nervous system) houses habitual and automatic impulses, archives our immortal life, and represents the sub-conscious (our past lives). The second part, cortex motor (the intermediary zone), is the motor to our human energy system, where effort and freewill reside. This is the conscious part of the being (our present life), where our present noble qualities (which we are currently edifying) are being stored. And lastly, the area of the brain which is least known by science and researchers, the frontal lobes, houses superior notions (ideals and superior goals) and the materials of our sublime order which are gradually conquered by our efforts for spiritual ascension; the super-conscious, the future – the area which allows the human mind to preview the future.

The human mind responsible for translating the contents of the soul with all its baggage from past lives, and its perspective of the future, helps in the construction of the individual's present reality, signaling the entire thought, emotional and physiological processes as a total expression of the soul's evolutionary condition, and thus establishes a direct spiritual dimension with the patient's health and well-being.

As illustrated in Dr. Carlos Alberto Jacob's methods, a patient's treatment depends on one of three probable causes of illness: "problems in one's current life, "karmic" problems from a past life, and problems originating in the spirit world or in the client's spiritual development. In the first instance, his treatment may include allopathic and homeopathic medicine, acupuncture, and/or conventional psychotherapy. In the second instance, past-life therapy is needed. In the third instance, spiritual exercises (for example exorcism, magnetic passes, "chakra cleansing," mediumship training) are required" (Krippner, 1987, p. 287). According to this diagnostic model, thought, feelings, and emotions imprinted on the soul have definite and direct influence on health and illness.

Pain and suffering of the physical body is only transitory; it is moral suffering that serves as a catalyst of spiritual evolution – an etiological agent rarely considered by classic medicine.

6

THE HUMAN ENERGY SYSTEM AND THE ROLE OF EMOTIONS IN HEALTH

It is always a difficult task to crystallize a concept that cannot be tangibly seen or touched by any of the human senses. This has been the case when dealing with explaining energy imbalances and therapies to patients. To understand the transferring of energies used by healing mediums (through the incorporation of benevolent spirit entities), the complex understanding of the perispirit and the human energy fields, which protect the human body and give it essential life force, is required.

Modern physics has demonstrated matter is a form of energy. In philosophical terms, form without matter is energy. God being immaterial (form without matter) is also energy. Humans composed of energy contain a sophisticated human electromagnetic field, which provides essential life force that is in the early beginnings of scientific development.

These are important revelations for the field of science and medicine. Brazilians believe further studies of electromagnetic energy will lead physicists to the source of human electromagnetic energy. Physicists, knowing that electromagnetic energy requires a source in order for it to function, are helping science gain a greater understanding of the human energy system and its role in biological function.

Many healing and spiritual world traditions include principles of the human energy system in their medical repertoires. Many Brazilians too, have come to use similar principles. As a system of inner and external light energy, the human energy field, comprises an aura: the fluctuating egg-shaped energy field that externally surrounds the body; and seven chakras: the spinning wheels of lights in the human body that function as vortices of energy. Think of the chakras as the human system of inner light. The aura and the chakras work systematically via a network of fine energy channels in the body called meridians.

Essential life-energy flows through the human being via these centers; when blockages occur in the channels it causes illness. Both information and light energy flows from the cosmos through the aura, into the chakras, filtered through the meridians. This is how the spirit world inspires us, and how light reaches the body cells, giving them potential life-sustaining energy. Each of the energy fields has a particular function and influences various emotional, mental, and physical (physiological) processes.

According to Barbara Ann Brennan in her book *Hands of Light: A Guide to Healing Through the Human Energy Field* (1987), she describes energy events within the auric field as always preceding the physical events. Her findings support a need for more energy healers to detect disease early on before a full manifestation of the illness occurs. Furthermore, it is essential to maintain a balanced functioning of the auric field to maintain optimal health. Her books are highly recommended to anyone wishing to further expand on the details of the human energy field thoroughly as it relates to issues of health and illness.

Each of the seven corresponding levels of energy found in the aura, has its own density and frequency. Each successive level becomes a higher frequency. The three major auras (the external layers of light surrounding the body) are visible to healers. In order from the layer furthest from the physical body, these are: the spiritual, mental, and etheric auras. The spiritual aura extends the farthest from the physical body, and has the highest frequency. Within the spiritual aura is the mental aura. Energy that is transmuted into mental energy appears in the mental aura – it reflects the mental state of a person. The final aura, the etheric (closest to the physical body, extends about eight inches from the body) reflects the emotional and physical health of a person, as it is the one that receives transmuted energy from the mental aura.

The aura expresses the qualities of a real man, it is the totality of his forces and emotions. It reveals the level of his spiritual development, mental capabilities and emotional nature, his state of well being, or state of illness, and his overall character. The aura being the energetic aspect of the human body is charged with a life force that vibrates with cosmic elements when it is in harmony.

As disease begins in the outer layers, energy fields lose their vibrancy. The physical body being the one with the lowest frequency reflects the disharmony that has formed into dense energy. If abuse of excessive alcohol, drugs or unclean living has occurred, the energy fields become dense, weakened, can be attacked, and can attract undesirable (spirit) attachments.

A more lucid explanation of "attachments" is given by Schwimmer in Robert Estrich-Pellegrino's book, *The Miracle Man*. "Look on an attached spirit as we would bacterium. When we are healthy, our immune system takes care of even deadly bacterium. When our immune system is weakened or damaged, then bacteria or viruses enter to create havoc. The same can be said for spirit attachment. If one's energy field is healthy and strong, spirits will not be able to enter" (p. 87).

Negative perceptions and emotions such as anger, rage, envy, greed, sadness, resentment, hate, vanity, intolerance, bitterness, pride, hypocrisy, fears, and even fanatic religiosity, being definite forms of energy, play a fundamental role in the creation of blocked energies. A curse, a bad thought, feeling, emotion, word, or action, is poison to the individual soul, poisoning every atom. Poisonous thoughts and emotions produce discordant tones, inharmony, and illness.

Negative feelings consuming a great deal of vital energy consequently in the process of energetic metabolism, create larger amounts of unhealthy, wasted energy. When the production of these negative energies exceeds the capacity of distribution and elimination, it accumulates in a corresponding organ or chakra, thus clogging vital energy in important energy terminals, creating fertile ground for the beginning of the physical disease process.

Ignoring the fact that individuals absorb and emit energy at all times through their thoughts, words, and actions has not allowed classic medicine to consider the symbiotic aspect of human energy, thoughts, and emotions in the pathological disease process. By dismissing the soul's influence over individual behavior, classic medicine's effort to modify human temperament and ill emotions has yet to be supported before the moral dispositions of the spirit. This may explain why efforts by classic medicine to modify human temperament have failed.

Spiritual knowledge leads to greater control of conflictive and explosive situations and has a positive effect on how these are dealt with. Spiritual knowledge also helps defeat one's own interior demons of *avarice* (selfishness, power, and pride), *pleasure* (of abusive eating, drinking, sex, and drugs), *anger* (aggression, vengeance, violence and hatred), *dejection* (mental depression), *accidie* (indifference, moral flab), and *kenodocila* (vanity, arrogance, presumptuousness). Spiritual knowledge teaches one to discipline and control one's senses and emotions.

When illness is present, balancing the patient's chakras should promote rapid healing and recovery. Harmonizing any imbalance can be done through a "realignment" of energy through a crystal bed therapy, (explained in the treatment modality section, chapter 11), and/or an astral infusion of essential divine energy, which provides a type of "boost" that reactivates the ill organism. This type of energy transfer can only be done through a healing medium, who as a human conduit enables a patient to receive a humanly adjusted dose of divine energy, only after having reduced the strength to human capacity.

Just as an electrical transformer is a conduit that reduces powerful voltage before entering a building with weaker voltage capacity, a healing medium is an efficient and effective conduit of divine energy for patients needing help with their electromagnetic spiritual framework.

PART THREE

SOUL DOCTORS, SOUL CLINICS, AND SOUL TREATMENT

7

SOUL DOCTORS, SOUL CLINICS:
THE SACRED MISSION OF HEALING MEDIUMS

Brazilian spiritists believe therapy for the soul requires soul doctors, soul clinics, the assistance of benevolent and highly evolved spirits, and a key treatment modality: *soul knowledge*. Immortal knowledge is obtained by cultivating faith, love, compassion, and discernment. In therapeutic terms this requires the patient be actively engaged in constant improvement of his/her morality, directly influencing all areas of their private and public life. The individuals whom have been entrusted with care of the human soul are healing mediums.

A sensorial perception function, *mediumship* is a condition by which relations between men and spirits is established. It is a natural human faculty, inherent to all human beings, at different levels and types. It is the attunement between an incarnate (living) and disincarnate (non-living) being that allows an adequate channel for perception of thoughts, will, and sentiments. This faculty may appear in any person regardless of the religious doctrine he/she embraces.

Great mediums of all creeds and from all times have been revealed; going as far back to the most ancient civilizations, including many related in the Bible. Their finality has been above all: an opportunity to serve, a blessing by which God has allowed humanity to maintain contact with the spiritual world. It is through His Word and mediumship that man has been able to be conscious of his immortal spiritual responsibilities.

Christ acknowledging the reality of a spirit world, taught humanity about secret doctrines. In the *Aquarian Gospel* we read, "Forbid not any man to do the works of God. There is no man who can pronounce the sacred Word, and in the name of Christ restore the sick and cast the unclean spirits out, who is not child of God ...The man of who you speak is one with us. Whoever gathers in the grain of heaven is one of us" (Dowling, 1979, p. 190). Mediums fulfill a sacred mission. They are specialists in the sacred and masters of spirit.

Healing mediums are not supposed to promise a cure, nor give false hope. Their mission is to put patients back on track with their spirituality, reconnecting them with the spirit world. If needed they can help identify a patient's obsessor, attempt dis-obsession procedures, minister passes, and provide fluidic magnetized water (energized with the healer's energy), all which contribute to reactivating the patient's own cure. Mediumistic healing practices as unorthodox and controversial as they may initially appear, have never contradicted the gospel teachings of Christ, nor have they opposed working collaboratively with allopathic medicine.

The following selection explains healing mediumship as a influential treatment modality. From the lesson of Udraka, among the sudras and visyas, the life and works of Jesus in India, illuminated in *The Aquarian Gospel of Jesus the Christ; the lost eighteen years so strangely silent in the New Testament*, a period Christ spent traveling and sharing wisdom with the masters, seers, and wise men in the temples and schools of Tibet, Egypt, India, Persia, and Greece:

"The healer is the man which can inspire faith. The tongue may speak to human ears, but souls are reached by souls that speak to souls .... He is the forceful man whose soul is large, and who can enter into souls, inspiring hope in those who have no hope, and faith in those who have no faith in God, in nature, nor in man ... A thousand things produce inharmony and make men sick; a thousand things may tune the harpsichord, and make men well .... That which is medicine for one is poison for another one; so one is healed by what would kill another one .... The virtue from the hand or breath may heal a thousand more; but love is queen. Thought, reinforced by love, is God's greatest sovereign balm ..... But many of the broken chords in life, and discords that so vex the soul, are caused by evil spirits of the air that men see not; that lead men on through ignorance to break the laws of nature and of God ...These powers act like demons, and they speak; they rend the man; they drive him to despair. ..... But he who is healer, true, is master of the soul, and can, by force or will, control these evil ones .... Some Spirits of the air are master spirits and are strong, too strong for human power alone; but man has helpers in the higher realms that may be importuned, and they will help to drive the demons out. .... Of what this great physician said, this is the sum. And Jesus bowed his head in recognition of the wisdom of this master soul, and went his way" (Dowling, 1979, pp. 58-59).

In Gadara, Jesus expelled unclean spirits out of a man. People in fear, believed that if He could drive the unclean spirits out, and being a man of such transcendent power, He could devastate their land at will, so they asked him to leave. Fear alone, leads people to resist and reject such powerful force.

Mediumship is a vocation and a God-given gift that requires to be practiced in a sacred and devout manner. "If there's one type of mediumship that demands this attitude more absolutely than the others, it is healing" (Kardec, 2000, p. 306-307). The healing medium in relaying healing energies, through good spirits channeling Divine energy, can never charge for his service. As Jesus told his disciples, "Heal the sick, raise the dead, cleanse those who have leprosy, drive out demons. Freely you have received, freely give" (Matthew, 10:8).

"God gave these gifts to them in order to ease other's suffering and to spread the faith. So Jesus told His disciples not to commercialize their gifts, i.e., to use them to earn profits or make a living" (Kardec, 2000, p 303). "Where there is no profit to be made, deceit is unlikely" (Kardec, 2000, p. 19). Besides its misuse is subject to Divine accountability. "... those endowed with this gift will have to account for the use to which they have put it, since they only received it in order to do good to their fellow human beings" (Kardec, 2000, p 333). Cultivating mediumship therefore requires a sincere disposition to serve.

8

ABADIANIA'S HEALING PHENOMENON: JOÃO DE DEUS

John of God, or João de Deus as he is affectionately called, is among the most powerful mediumistic healers existing at the present time. João has worked as a healing, physical, and unconscious, medium for almost five decades at the Casa de Dom Inácio, in the small town of Abadiania, in central Brazil. This healing phenomenon is fulfilling his sacred mission of serving humanity by setting an example and providing a new model of medicine for the rest of the world. "I do not heal anyone – God alone is the healer," João continuously answers to the never-ending expressions of gratitude from the multitudes he has treated while in-entity.

João is in his sixties now and has been healing since he was a teenager. He has devoted his life to healing the sick, and provides his service free of charge or will lose his gift. He embodies more than thirty spirit entities who perform "miraculous" healings on those who seek him, and those whom God merits a cure. He does not remember anything about the events that take place while he is "incorporated" by a benevolent spirit, yet the fact remains that many have been cured of serious health problems under his care.

Many of these patients have been diagnosed with terminal and incurable diseases. The entities working through Divine intervention, and through João as the vessel, have cured every type of cancer, AIDS, muscular dystrophy, asthma, multiple sclerosis, heart disease, stroke complications, blindness, and paralysis. João in entity is a master of de-possession, treating the cursed, witched, and insane. He has accomplished wonders with patients suffering from depression, drug and alcohol addictions. He has been tested and studied by scientists and physicians who have concluded no fraud is involved, although they find no comfortable explanation to his work within the current and soloist scientific paradigm.

[*Images on the right: Clockwise, starting with the upper right photo: João in entity doing a visible spiritual surgery in front of the crowd; an image of Christ on the casa wall taken while a spiritual surgery was taking place; the line outside the casa of patients waiting for a consultation with João in entity; the line inside the current room of patients walking through on their way to see João in entity; João in entity addressing the crowd; center photo: João in entity doing a visible spiritual surgery on a patient in front of the casa crowd. His assistant, Dr. Uehara a medico-espírita from Sao Paulo*].

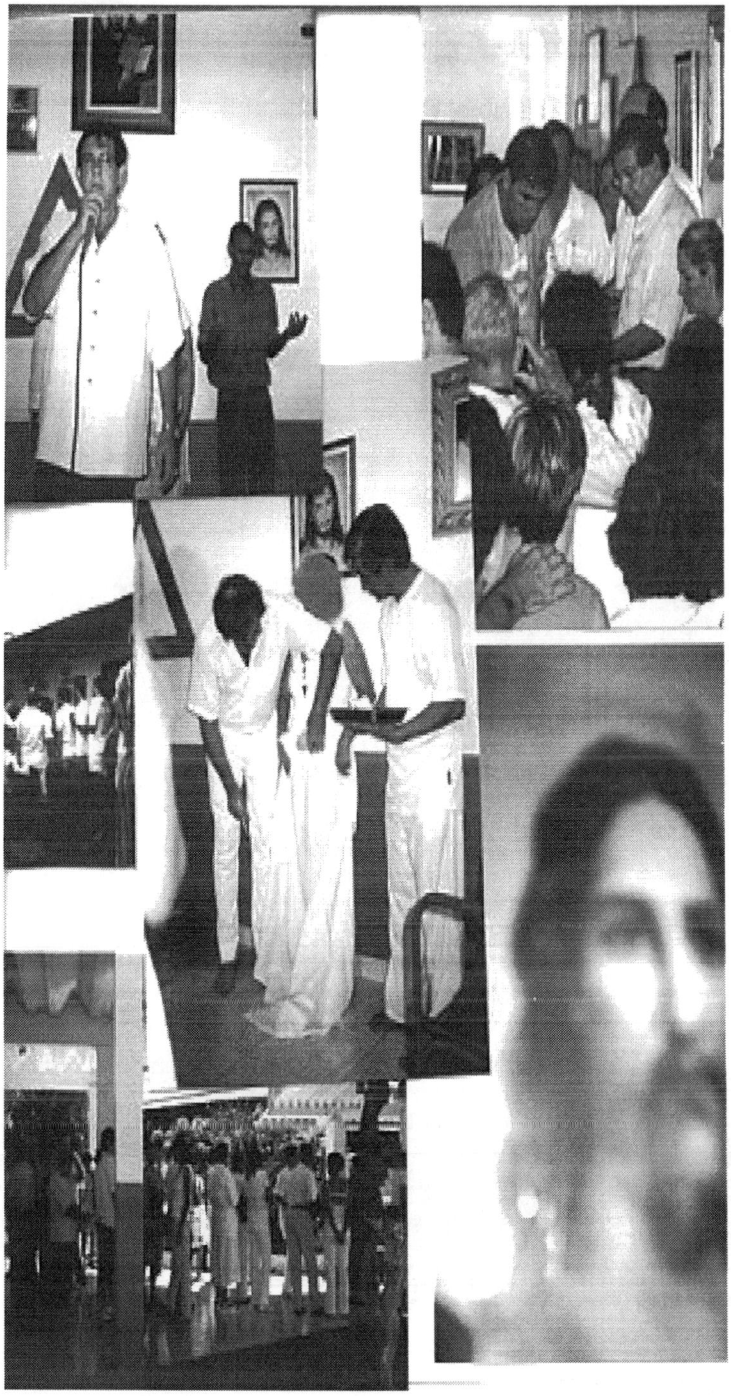

João has dedicated his life to humanity. His purpose in life is to heal the sick and to make people aware that we are here on earth to improve our level on the "other side," to elevate and better the position of of the soul in the hereafter by what it does in this physical life (Estrich-Pellegrino, 1997). At the young age of sixteen, "he accepted the responsibility of devoting his life to spirit incorporation for the purpose of healing the sick. He accepted a lifelong task that would demand much of him and frequently repay him with abuse, personal deprivation, persecution, and unlawful incarceration" (Estrich-Pellegrino, p. 6).

John of God is a humble and devoutly God-loving man. He accepts and treats all without prejudice or religious bias. Personally belonging to a society (the U.S.) that does not have an equal distribution of health resources or access, this genuine type of healthcare delivery system is justly commendable. João heals the poor just in the same manner that he heals the rich or famous and receives no payment for his services. He is a model example of a genuine and effective healing medium.

"His purpose in life is to heal the sick and to make people aware that we are here on earth to improve our level on the "other side." To elevate and better the position of the soul in the hereafter by what it does in this physical life." – Estrich Pellegrino

João has been endowed with faith, filled with goodwill, and understanding of the spirit's predominance over the physical (material) world. Most importantly, João and other genuine healing mediums teach their patients to act on internal direction and to learn to discriminate between thoughts motivated by strength and patience (faith) and those by fear and illusion (which characterize human weakness).

Strength and patience are necessary for healing to occur, particularly if the healing does not occur instantaneously. Strength, courage, and wisdom are needed to understand that the Lord has his own reasons for healing one person instantly and another over a period of time.

At the Casa de Dom Inácio the entities that João incorporates are benevolent spirits of deceased physicians, surgeons, healers, psychologists, and theologians, who cite God as the only healing source. Through João as the medium or vessel, the disincarnate entities (spirits) assist him with the diagnosis and treatment of those who are ill and make the long journey to the small town. At this healing sanctuary, conventional medical physicians, and Brazilian allopathic Spiritist doctors (*Médico-Espiritas*), assist healing-medium João while learning from the greater realms of medicine.

These partnerships (healers, spirits, and doctors) are seen throughout the many healing sanctuaries in Brazil. Serving as both sanctuaries and healthcare facilities, *casas and centros* provide patients with comprehensive medical care. Patients report the attention to be more personal, compassionate, effective, and efficient.

9

CASA DE DOM INÁCIO: A MULTI-FAITH NON-DENOMINATIONAL HEALING SANCTUARY: TREATS WOUNDED AND FLABBY SOULS

The *casa* plays a unique role in reaffirming people's faith of a greater power to patients, healers and doctors alike. A multi-functional facility that satisfies the needs of the mind, soul and body, all in one place and houses a unique collaboration of multidisciplinary therapies, all in one location. The casa provides a healing environment conducive to patients of all walks of life, social strata, creeds, and nationalities. The participation of the community in a patients healing means that the sick individual receives a great deal of social support from family, and friends (incarnate and disincarnate).

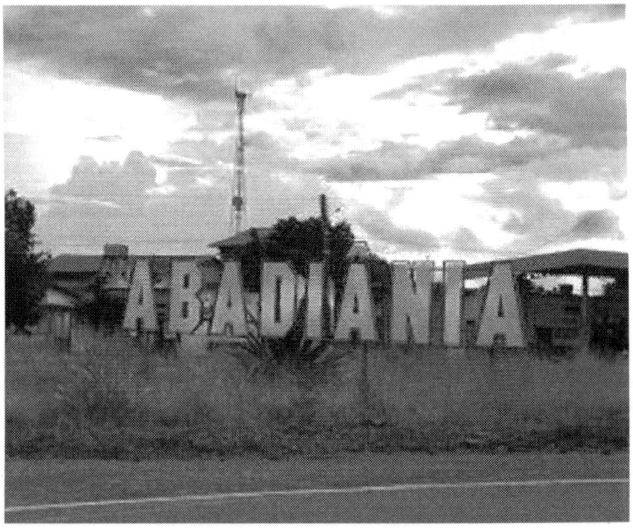

Abadiania, central Brazil

Unlike a conventional clinical treatment plan, a treatment that also accommodates the patients spiritual needs, should deal more effectively with any prior moral transgressions. For those who lack an arduous self-discipline or may have forgotten the basic human principles and feel the need of a mentor that can work with them in their relationship with God, the medium as spiritual advisor can help accomplish this.

The *casa's* simple and non-bureaucratic nature saves the patient a tremendous amount of unneeded frustration and aggravation that is typical of the complex organization found in most conventional settings. To begin, there are no patient-referral prerequisites, or prolonged waiting periods awaiting authorization or insurance verification – requirements that only extend the already exhaustive treatment process for a patient, which must have an effect on health outcomes.

There is no patient-billing department required to bill, and collect accounts from patients and third-party payors. A *casa's* multidisciplinary aspect (containing all medical specialties in one facility) eliminates the generation of separate bills for the variety of medical providers used in diagnostic and treatment procedures (e.g., radiology, anesthesiology, laboratory, specialty consultations, etc.), thus eliminating many unnecessary frustrations and added costs. Sounds like something from out of this world, but it is the reality of *the casas* in Brazil.

The *casa* also serves as a teaching institution for healthcare professionals as well as for individuals. For health practitioners it provides education and training that was excluded from conventional medical school curriculums. Thus, such an educational experience offers a new perception that takes health professionals beyond the pathological and physiochemical analysis of the human body, to explore a missing component in medicine, the human soul.

The setting, and the collaborative environment found at the *casa* is teaching western-trained doctors that medicine is an expression of compassion (literally in action), one that is applied to all facets of this most noble and humble vocation, and begins with a fundamental transformation of the patient-doctor relationship.

By unlearning and re-educating health professionals, they understand new values that increase the patient's responsibility in their own care. This is helping physicians learn the importance of cultivating a reciprocal trusting relationship with their patients. *The casa* serves as an important research center that unites a variety of academic disciplines conducting investigations. Archives of daily videos, patient records, and testimonials are kept and are available to researchers, healthcare professionals, skeptics, and the general public.

> *"Unlike a conventional clinical treatment plan, a treatment that also accommodates the patients spiritual needs, should deal more effectively with any prior moral transgressions."*

As a school for other, non-healthcare individuals (patients or visitors), *casas* provide what an educational, medical, and religious institution offer: knowledge, treatment, health and spiritual advise, respectively. Rather than to deal with various institutions, the casa accommodates the patient's multidisciplinary needs all under the same roof. An ill mind, or a diseased body is being treated while the soul is being cared for.

As a non-profit healthcare facility, a *casa* fully operated by a voluntary staff offers a place where individuals can participate in such a gratifying experience. Working with patients whose conditions are grave helps volunteers see their sometimes ungrateful, indifferent, unforgiving, and unfaithful dispositions, as trivial.

While doctors, patients, and visitors compose most of the demographic makeup of the *casa*, members of the paranormal international (as well as national) community also represent a significant population group. Genuine members of the paranormal community have an important mission of removing barriers between humankind and the spirit realm. They are the delegated guardians of sacred wisdom. In this respect the *casa* is not only a teaching institution for doctors, patients and visitors. It also serves as the site for potential mediums to receive inspiration, training, and guidance. In serving as transcendental teaching institutions for future generations of healing mediums and *medico-espiritas*, the Casa de Dom Inácio as well as other *casas* are helping new generations of integrative health professionals who will complete the monumental work of transcendental medicine.

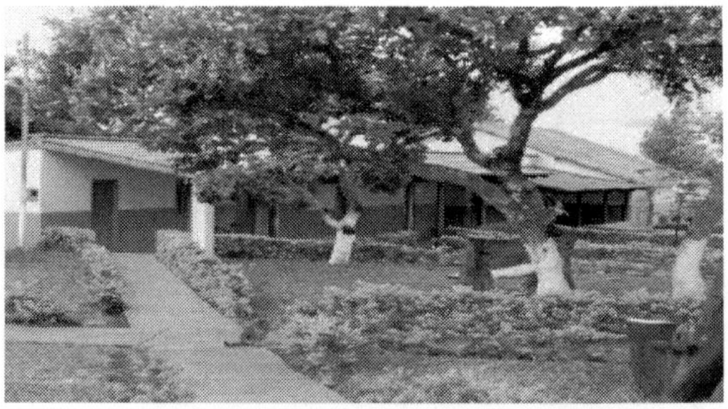

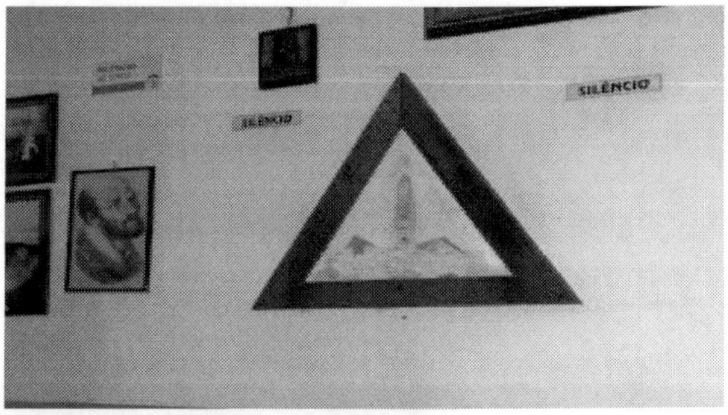

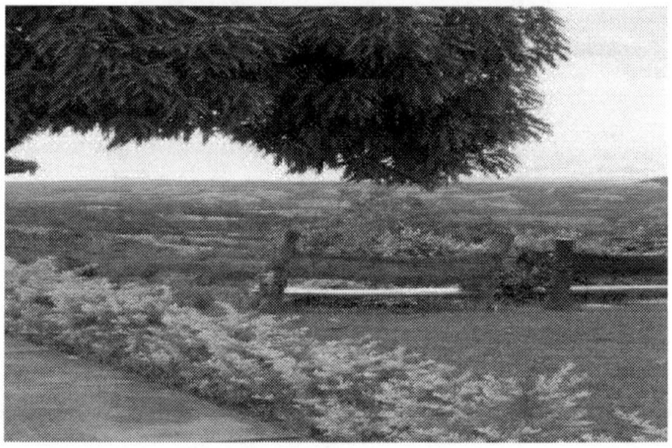

The serene grounds at the Casa de Dom Inácio

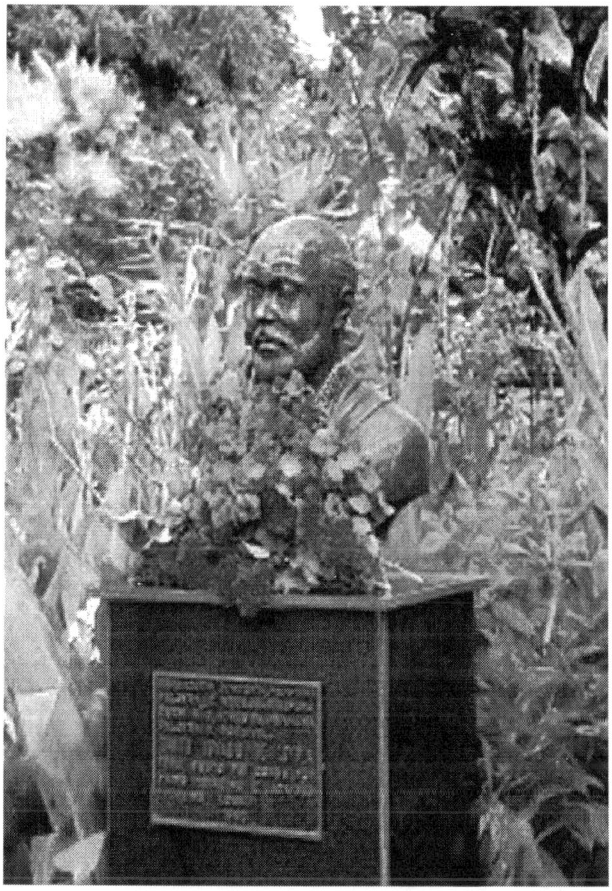

Casa garden dedicated to
St. Ignatius

10

PATRON ENTITY OF THE CASA DE DOM INÁCIO: SAINT IGNATIUS DE LOYOLA

The interfaith aspect of the Casa de Dom Inácio in Abadiania, Brazil, is a most profound aspect of the healing that goes on there. The casa respects everyone, all creeds; all of God's children come together as one. All drawing from the same source, praying together, with one thought, one heart, for one family, one God – an incredible healing experience.

It was world-renowned medium, Chico Xavier, who requested João de Deus name the casa after the founder of the Jesuit Order, Santo Ignacio de Loyola, and selected Abadiania as the site for the new casa.

Ignatius de Loyola was a great defender and soldier of Christ and His Church. His heart and his passion for the Glory of God is translated in his struggles of faith and justice, in the relationship between faith and cultures, and in the inter-religious dialogue that has at it's depth an intimate experience with God. This could explain why he continues his work from the spirit realm, in embracing the wider community and directing this multi-faith healing sanctuary in central Brazil.

St. Ignatius of Loyola founded the Society of Jesus, better known as the Jesuit Order of the Catholic Church in 1540. This order is characterized by its moral education and intellectual contributions, primarily at colleges and universities, as well as missionary work and ministry of human rights and social justice. Most strikingly, the Jesuit's education encourages a study of all the major world religions in order that their students can identify the thread of continuity between them – that of a higher power.

During this time period in his hometown of Azpeitia, Spain, as well as through most of Europe, European society had been challenged by ideas of Humanism and Renaissance – both significantly characterized by the importance of knowledge. As he grew stronger in faith and discipline, he found this knowledge in pursuing a Christian education and taking it to all parts of the globe, with his ministry that reached Brazil in the 16th century.

In his attempt to save and gather souls for the kingdom of Christ he authored *The Spiritual Exercises* that remain instrumental in the spiritual life of many today, and left his immortal works of the Jesuit Order to grow in numbers and in faith. Members of the new order, dedicated themselves to the teachings of a Christian education, with all the beauty revealed in the form of sacred art. The Society of Jesus dispersed the teachings of Christ and put the love of Jesus into action as they set out to carry His name and His Word to foreign lands. While Inácio reached the Glory of God with his immortal works, his earlier days, prior to his

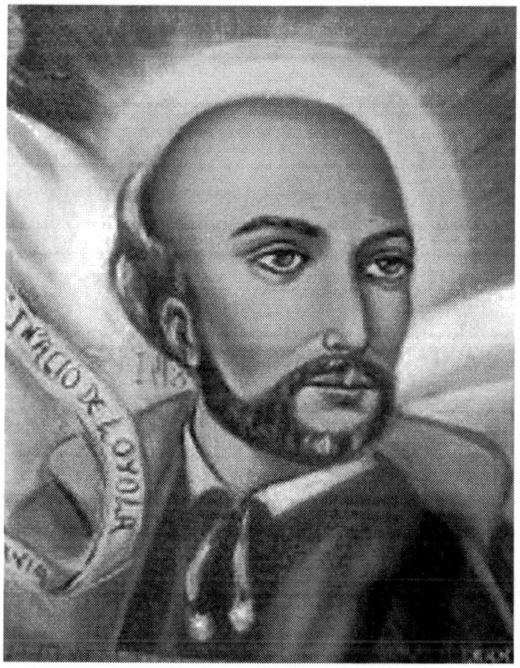

Patron Entity of the Casa De Dom Inácio
St. Ignatius de Loyola

re-awakening, were of a young and rebellious heart.

Born December 24, 1491 to a very rich and noble family, Ignacio was the last child born to a very large family (some sources say the family had thirteen children, others claim there were eleven). He grew into a violent and aggressive young man. His reawakening occurred after he was wounded in battle against the French at Navarro. He and his men were captured by French troops but his great courage and valor, being quite impressive, earned Ignacio and his men their release. He went into a coma and received a vision from Peter, the Apostle, who healed his wounded leg and advised him to change his ways.

Later Ignacio would receive a vision of the Blessed Mother of God, who inspired him to write the

Spiritual Exercises, the spiritual manual of how to get rid of all human attachments to get the soul closer to Christ. These spiritual exercises are an open invitation for everyone to participate in a profound experience with the Mystery of God, which ultimately is the only experience that will give life true meaning. The exercises involve a four-week program that starts with the full examination of conscience: an exam of thoughts, words, and deeds and recommends it be followed with a confession and Holy Communion (an important catholic ritual that refers to taking the Sacred Eucharist, or the Body and Blood of Christ, something Christ instructed His disciples to do in His memory).

Week two is the deep contemplation of the two standards, those of Christ, and those of Satan. It is about the contemplation of the nature of good and evil. Or as Jesus would of described it in Aramaic, the contemplation of a ripened seed and one that is not yet ripened.

Week three takes the soul through contemplation at midnight. It reviews eating rules and goes over the types of prayer, such as reading scripture, meditation, contemplation, adoration and praise, and petitioning a specific request or blessing.

Week four is to relive the mysteries of the life, passion, death, and resurrection of Christ. During this week, one also learns the rules for the discernment of spirits: through both, spiritual consolation (positive and superior spirits influencing us, the light of the soul), and spiritual desolation (negative and lowly spirits influencing our thoughts; the darkness of the soul). After becoming acquainted with his Spiritual Exercises it is clear why St. Ignatius was named the patron saint of spiritual retreats, and why he is invoked for protection against negative spirits.

The Blessed Mother of Christ advised him to travel and teach the way of light. He listened and resigned to all of his worldly possessions, which coming from a very wealthy family meant giving up a substantial amount of material goods, status, and prestige. He went as far as to exchange his fine clothes with that of a beggar. He traveled by foot through Spain en route to Jerusalem stopping at the altar of Our Lady of Montserrate, outside of Barcelona. He was ridiculed, persecuted, and eventually became gravely ill.

His stop outside of Barcelona, in Manresa, turned into a 10-month stop. Here he fasted, prayed and read for hours every day. It is here where he experienced a vision and joyous exaltation (levitation), which happened during the time that he was praying. He would go into a mystical trance that caused a light to radiate from his forehead.

It is also during this time that he read the *Imitation of Christ* by T. Kempes, which he would then carry with him for daily meditation. Ignacio gained profound mystical knowledge of the Trinity, God's Act of Creation, the presence of Christ in the Eucharist, and the Humanity of Christ and Mary. He was further inspired by reading "Lives of the Saints," particularly those of Assisi, Antonio de Padua, and Dominic. Ignacio taught many how to find peace of soul, but he was imprisoned for these teachings as he was accused of having no ecclesiastical validity.

In 1528 he set out to Paris to finish his studies. He is there seven years. Here his spiritual exercises follow the formula of a retreat, calling for a complete withdrawal from the world for a month of solitude, prayer, and meditation. Spiritual reflection, distanced from worldly distractions, is an integration of the self in order to discover how to enter into communion with God, under the standards of Christ.

In a remote church outside of Rome, God the Father and His Son showed themselves to Ignacio, telling him "We shall see you favored by Rome," and so the Society of Jesus received rigorous examination and approval by Pope Paul III, who admitted the will of God and confirmed the Society, on August 15, 1534.

"Spiritual reflection, distanced from worldly distractions, is an integration of the self in order to discover how to enter into communion with God, under the standards of Christ."

Ignacio was blessed with the healing power of God as he used his gift to free a possessed girl of evil sprits by making the sign of the cross. Another time, he healed a good friend who was dying, by embracing him. His passion however was to sermon the crowds with the Word of God in order to save souls for the kingdom of heaven. He paid a hefty price for this. His love for Christ and his prayerful devotion to saving souls for the kingdom of God, often times was met with him being tormented by demons and lowly spirits who saw him as waging a spiritual war.

Naming the Casa after Ignacio de Loyola, a penitent sinner turned saint, who after experiencing a complete spiritual reawakening and surrendering completely and wholeheartedly to God, and who became one of the most influential spiritual figures in Christian history, gives the Casa de Dom Inácio, his great warrior spirit.

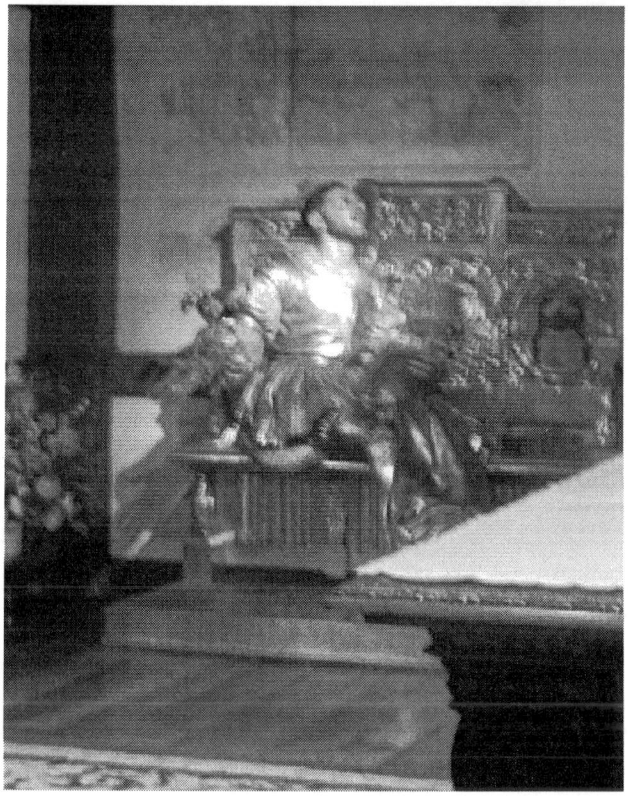

St. Ignatius' room where he surrendered to God, Azpeitia, Spain

SURRENDER

by St. Ignatius Loyola

Lord Jesus Christ, take away my freedom, my memory, my understanding, and my will. All that I have and cherish; all that You have given me. I surrender it all to be guided by Your will. Your love and Your grace are wealth enough for me. Give me these, Lord Jesus, and I ask for nothing more. Amen.

Anima Christi

(SOUL OF CHRIST)

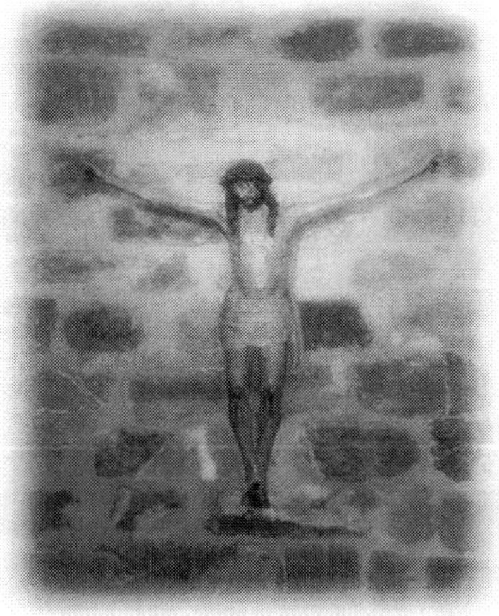

Soul of Christ, sanctify me
Body of Christ, save me.
Blood of Christ, inebriate me.
Water from the side of Christ, wash me.
Passion of Christ, strengthen me.
O good Jesus, hear me.
Within Thy wounds shelter me.
Separated from Thee, let me never be.
From the malignant enemy defend me.
And bid me come to Thee.
That with Thy saints I may praise Thee
Forever and ever. Amen

An indulgence of 300 days.

An indulgence of 7 years,
if recited after Holy Communion.

- St. Ignatius Loyola

11

NON-SURGICAL TREATMENT MODALITIES AND REGIMENS

Interestingly, *none* of the non-surgical treatment modalities used in spiritual healing are utilized in the traditional biomedical model. Marked by impersonalization, the classic model at the present time uses *maintenance*-oriented care (only suppresses symptoms but may not necessarily heal them), and when needed, a prescription drug regimen that tends to be mostly suppressive in nature, rather than curative.

Spiritual healers, characterized by a high degree of personalization, believe the only way for a patient to achieve integral healing is by activating the patient's soul that allows important spiritual, emotional, mental, and physiological processes to take place. The spiritual model may include a natural drug therapy that treats the cause of the disease (not just suppress symptoms) thus activates self-healing properties, while stressing a more *prevention*-oriented care regimen that involves more than just changing diet, exercise, abusive and harmful habits. This model extends to prevention-oriented care that should include modifying ones personal code of ethics and moral conduct.

Activating the soul is done by diagnosing the patient's ailment with a spiritual consultation, where the healing medium reads the patient's electromagnetic spiritual framework: the aura, chakras, mind, soul, and body, ultimately detecting any energy and spiritual imbalance. A healing medium (such as João de Deus) can see beyond the patient's physical body (the patient's soul), to also read a blueprint of the patient's past incarnations and can detect whether illness originated from a spiritual imbalance in this lifetime, or if it is karmic (from past existences). [This is not to be misinterpreted. Not all ill conditions or individual suffering indicate a person has bad karma that needs atonement. Sometimes different problems may be disguised, to take the patient to a reawakening of the soul, to higher studies, to more knowledge and experiences that will also contribute to the patient's evolutionary progress].

At the Casa de Dom Inácio, healer João de Deus in conducting spiritual consultations, examines the spiritual framework of the ill patient, and identifies the source of the ailment. Rather than to use biomedical diagnostic equipment or technology to diagnose and treat a patient's physical condition, João gives a spiritual examination, and recommends a treatment plan that not only alleviates the physical symptoms, but also addresses the *cause* of the condition.

Depending on the individual case, healers may also recommend the patient be simultaneously treated with conventional biomedical treatment. Spiritual healing may be complementary to other treatments, rather than an alternate source (as is the case with alternative medicine).

Reenergizing a patient's energy system may be the initial step involved in the patients healing process. If the healing medium, such as João, upon his spiritual consultation, identifies an imbalance or a weak aura or energy system, João (in entity) will prescribe either a crystal bed treatment, or ask the patient to sit in "current" and meditate; or will recommend (visible or invisible) surgical intervention. This latter therapeutic intervention will be described in a following section.

The crystal bed treatment allows the patient to lay on a bed (face up) while receiving energy from seven crystal lights that are aligned with the patient's seven chakras - energy centers - while listening to smooth, relaxing music and receiving a bath of celestial energy. At the end of the crystal bath session, the patient's energy is balanced and energized. With a realigned and reenergized electromagnetic spiritual framework, the patient having received a type of perispirit adjustment now has realigned, unclogged, and improved the condition to his means of spiritual communication. Once treated a patient's extra-sensorial channels should allow for optimal performance in the flow of energy between the patient and cosmos.

A patient at this point has been prepped and is now ready to undergo intensive therapeutic intervention utilizing an essential educational regimen that proposes a new type of learning system, having the potential to reach the depths of the individual soul with the incredible ability to induce personal change and transformation. This type of education is not necessarily found within the usual boundaries of an institution or a classroom, nor one found in an already existing curriculum, instead it is one that goes with the individual's own pace, desire, and motivation to learn.

Educating the soul involves an education that awakens human consciousness to potential values, goodness, altruism, and solidarity. It helps develop the positive human attributes originally planted within, but due to a host of reasons has either been neglected or forgotten, generating a type of moral flab or spiritual laziness, as St. Ignatius would of described it.

To treat moral flab, or spiritual laziness, patients must first learn to go beyond the "*I* and *Mine*" to the "*We* and *Ours/Theirs.*" Just as the physical body requires physical exercise, the flabby soul also requires disciplinary exercises to adhere to. A genuine soul education allows the individual to think critically, and appreciate the importance and significance of their human existence, and allows them to live with dignity, abundance, and purpose regardless of their unique social position.

Faith is both human and divine. It can be used to satisfy earthly needs or heavenly and future aspirations. It is where a person places their free-will at the service of divine force and inspiration, which often results in what is perceived as a miracle, when in reality, is nothing more than the development of a human gift given to all. Through faith, our human voyage of exploration, we can accomplish miracles of selfless love, and devotion. It is a most powerful tool in correcting any negative impulses of the soul, and has incredible power to release internal healing energy.

The positive and definite effects of prayer are also revealed in the "current" rooms at the Casa de Dom Inácio. The only prerequisite to enter these rooms is to be open to love, and to freely give before receiving God's grace. The rooms are filled with patients (including those who have exhausted all efforts with conventional medicine) who are involved in deep meditation and prayer where they receive divine inspiration, energy, and healing. This room is a place where emotions are felt at the deepest level, as if being in the presence of God.

> *"To treat moral flab, or spiritual laziness, patients must first learn to go beyond the "I and Mine" to the "We and Ours/Theirs."*

As Josie RavenWing so accurately describes in her book *The Book of Miracles: The Healing Work of João de Deus* (2002), "Within seconds I felt an overwhelming wave of energy pass through me that was of such a pure quality of Love that I dissolved into tears. The wave was warm, almost hot, like a flame passing through me and burning away all that was not love. I tried to keep from sobbing out loud so as not to disturb the others, but I felt like I was absolutely melted by this Love" (RavenWing, 2002, pp 25-26). This statement is by far the closest that expresses the sacredness of the healing experience at the Casa de Dom Inácio.

Aside from working with the energy system, João usually gives his patients an herbal remedy that includes a few minor dietary restrictions. While the entity that prescribes the individual remedy, blesses the prescription with powerful individual and personal spiritual properties that elicit the patient's healing, the herbal base prescribed and found in all the remedies is passionflower. Interestingly, there is also divine inspiration in the particular herb that is used in the patient's treatment.

The passionflower capsules have a unique component. "The healing power of a plant spirit medicine lies in their unique ability to evoke a sense of well-being in mind, body, and spirit. This quality springs from the natural affinity that exists between their energy and our own" (Harvey & Cochrane, 1999,

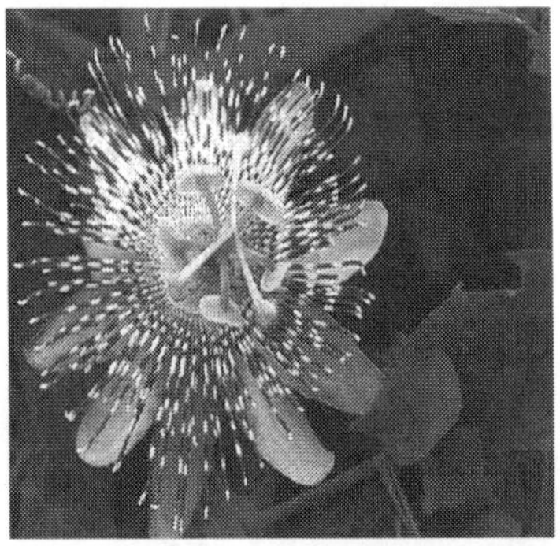

"I am the soul flower that holds the energy of divine consciousness. I help with the evolution of mankind."
- Harvey & Cochrane

p. 26). "Plants spirit medicines act as catalysts for rebalancing the body's energy. This is because each particular plant holds a special form of spirit energy that resonates with our own life force" (Harvey & Cochrane, p. 27). Although the herbal base is the same for all patients, passionflower, each prescription is provided with a specific spiritual blessing to treat the patient's particular condition. In Harvey & Cochrane's experience, *passiflora* (passionflower) has shown to be more than just a simple herbal remedy.

"I am the soul flower that holds the energy of divine consciousness. I help with the evolution of mankind." These flowers are best known for their tranquilizing properties, but their spirit inspires a more ethereal sense of the divine. This flower is identified closely to Jesus Christ – "the Spanish conquistadors, who compared the emergence of this beautiful blossom from its unassuming bud with the Passion of Christ. The flower's intricate patterns represent the five instruments of Christ's crucifixion: the hammer, spears, nails, crowns of thorns and pillar where he was lashed" (Harvey & Cochrane, 1999, p. 155). One can easily see how the spirit of this flower mirrors the divinity embodied by Jesus. "Attuning to it evokes a sense of compassion, altruism, and unconditional love ..... Passionflower also opens the heart and throat chakras to higher or more spiritual levels of consciousness" (Harvey & Cochrane, 1999, pg. 155). In addition the budding flower is purple, the same color that is symbolic of the Passion of Christ.

As a patient who took this remedy, I will add that this herbal prescription is quite unique, as it definitely has unique healing properties. For me particularly, it had the ability to amplify my love and compassion for others, unlike any other passionflower product I had taken before. I was very much aware of this while I was taking the remedy. My love for everyone was magnified, and the compassion I felt, especially for beggars on the streets, was inexplicable. There were times when I'd break out crying from seeing their unfortunate circumstances. Without a doubt, this herbal remedy allowed me to experience a higher level of spiritual consciousness, to attune to my greater self.

Aside from the passionflower herbal prescription, a patient's plan of treatment will involve hydrotherapy (involving both external and/or internal consumption). Water is important in purifying both the spiritual, and physical bodies, as it is an optimal conductor of electromagnetic force. During a healing session at the Casa de Dom Inácio it is customary for patients to drink as much fluidized water during their stay there. It is also encouraged to continue drinking this water at home. Many travel with cases of water back to their respective countries. João in entity turns regular drinking water into *fluidized water, with the healing energies he transmits to the water.*

For those unfamiliar with fluidized water, it is water that has been blessed or meditated upon, and has received heaven's medicinal balm through the radiations of the healer's best energies.

Fluidized water is also the custom at the Temple of Goodwill in Brasilia. The Legion of Goodwill in its publication by Jose de Paiva Netto, *"Spiritualistic Guidelines of the World LGW"* volume one (1989), Netto notes: Jesus is the shepherd of the ecumenical flock, of a true world fraternity headed by Jesus and directed by the LGW (Legion of Goodwill). Many governments from across the globe, as well as many religious dignitaries have honored this exemplary ecumenical temple.

The Temple of Goodwill also offers holy fluidic water for all who visit. A reprint of the Prayer of the Glass of Water, written by Alziro Zarur (founder of the LGW) was written more than 30 years ago, and can be found at the end of this book in the section of Brazilian Prayers.

The spiritual strength attached to this prayer can be best understood by the explanation Dr. Masaru Emoto gives, in his book *The Hidden Messages in Water*. In his book he demonstrates the spiritual consciousness of water that comes through the healing power of love and gratitude. A Japanese scientist, Emoto has made significant progress in the field of spiritual consciousness, by discovering molecules of water that are affected by human thoughts, words, and feelings. He has photographed the crystal formations created by different thought forms and words. When using words such as "love and gratitude," they formed beautiful crystals. While a negatively charged statement, such as "kill him," created ugly and distorted images, quite different from what a loving thought or positive phrase created. His work is irrefutably an eye opener for non-believers and skeptics alike.

The *cachoeira,* (a natural waterfall) which is only a few minutes away from the Casa de Dom Inácio, offers yet another type of hydrotherapeutic treatment. For those who João in entity prescribes a visit to the *cachoeira*, it is yet another way for patients to get reconnected with nature.

The waterfall is intended to be a sacred moment with nature and the spirit world, and not supposed to be used as a recreational getaway, nor a romantic hideaway. The casa has rules for patients to abide by during their visit there. It is advised that one become familiarized with the casa rules before visiting this wonderful, supernatural landscape.

Along with the prescribed hydrotherapy, and passionflower remedies, there may also be a few dietary restrictions to be followed, particularly, while taking the remedies. Patients are told to abstain from eating pork, pepper (spicy foods), and consuming alcohol while taking the herbal remedies. These dietary restrictions, the *casa* volunteers explain, aid the physical body in healing during the recovery process.

Being *open* to change becomes crucial in the process of integral healing. While social ills are considered non-physiological determinants of health, they have a direct negative effect on health. Many who over, or under eat do so to offset the emotional, ethical and spiritual distress in their lives.

Over or under eating (commonly associated to chronic stress), sleep deprivation (weakens lymphocytes), societal stress (affects the immune system and consequently morbidity and mortality), substance abuse (weakens the immune system), alcoholism (not only has tremendous adverse effects on health but also on the economy), and smoking (important risk factor to cardiovascular disease and lung cancer), can only be healed when the patient actively engages in seeking a pathway that will activate his own emotional, spiritual, and physical recovery.

"Being open to change becomes crucial in the process of integral healing."

Healing therefore involves a much more active role on behalf of the patient. Whereas a cure occurs when the *physical* progression of an illness has been *controlled*, it only alleviates symptoms temporarily as it does not deal with the emotional and psychological stresses that affected it; making it highly probable that the illness will recur. The patient while recovering temporarily and not having fully dealt emotionally or spiritually with the source of the illness, may never experience complete healing.

Emotional and spiritual recovery, is achieved only when a patient has gained a genuine desire to release all negative patterns, retrain, and reactivate it's human soul, emotions, and energy system.

Identifying negative emotions, ways of thinking and acting can help patients make the connection between their ill spiritual system and their ill physical symptoms. Educating and purifying the soul then becomes the pivotal treatment in the course of a patient's healing. Obtaining spiritual healing and consequently regaining physical health.

Regular meditation, prayer, and charitable works are essential to the healing process as they are essential elements in maintaining a state of spiritual equilibrium. Without activating this important internal power to heal, disease will continue to have its way with the physical body.

Faith and Prayer, according to Dr. Larry Dossey, author of *Healing Words* (1993) from a medical perspective is preventative medicine, capable of preventing sin and healing wrong. His research work has contributed to a growing number of US medical school courses that now teach the importance of spirituality in health.

Faith and prayer provide us with a guide to ethical living, teaching discipline, self-control, and the proper conformed emotional behavior. Together they constitute personal courage that aids a patient in becoming fully active in his personal transformation. Becoming active and self-responsible helps the individual find true purpose in life.

The importance of being strong in faith, hope, and love in order to protect the soul from harming or destroying itself is found in many of the different world spiritual traditions and teachings.

Fear being the opposite of faith, transgresses human trust in Divine guidance. Only faith and love can keep evil from penetrating the mind, soul, and body. By constantly wearing an armor of love and faith (through constant prayer) a vigilant and disciplined soul cannot be disturbed. When the soul has overcome obstacles of fear it has done so because it has learned to love, to forgive, to let go, to creatively express a new transformed self.

The mind when vibrating in elevated tonality, blocks the approximation of less evolved spirits and is more receptive to higher evolved spirit influences that positively affect human intelligence, and emotional behavior. There exists a reciprocal exchange between human beings and spiritual entities: humans acting upon spirit help (through prayer and through mental vibrations/frequencies), and highly evolved spirit entities acting equally upon humans (intuitively, clarifying, and orienting them) together labor towards the realization of good acts. By the same token, if the spirit world senses a vibrational tune that consists of negative thoughts or feelings, the lower evolved spirits can negatively influence the individual, causing him to do wrong, or bring the person a mental disturbance such as an obsession or mental subjugation.

There is growing scientific evidence to these energy vibrations. Amit Goswani, a world-recognized quantum physicist and author of *Physics of the Soul* (2001) is demonstrating that the presence of the subtle fields in the human electromagnetic structure allows us to receive the energy vibrations of prayers. He has also used concepts of quantum physics to give credence to metaphysical theories of reincarnation and immortality, and has successfully defined consciousness as the primary reality.

> *"Whereas a cure occurs when the physical progression of an illness has been controlled, it only alleviates symptoms temporarily as it does not deal with the emotional and psychological stresses that affected it; making it highly probable that the illness will recur."*

Faith, prayer, and meditation are the most prescribed therapies at these healing sanctuaries. It is in the *current rooms* that this most efficient and effective healing modality allows an exchange of divine inspiration and healing to take place. The intensity of divine light that is found in these sanctuaries helps activate the four white seeds of will, faith, love, and helpfulness. When these seeds are cultivated in humility, wisdom of impartiality, impermanence, and depth, the results can be incredible, what many call miraculous.

Fraternal love and solidarity being a human being's maximum conquest – is universal love put into

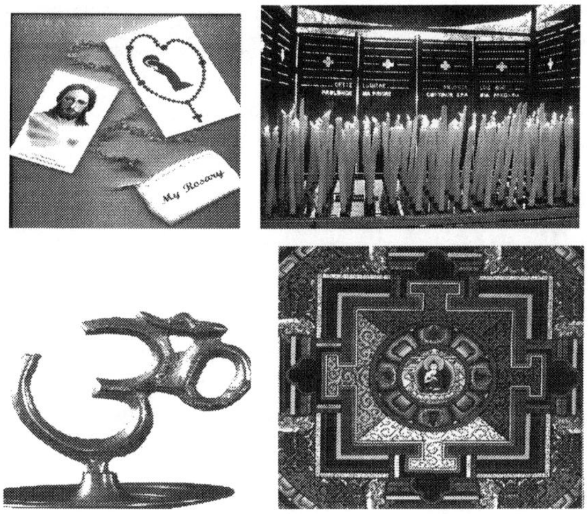

Sacred tools of worship: (clockwise) Prayer and the Holy Rosary; candle lighting conveys important messages to the heavens; the OM is the receptacle of Supreme Truth; a meditative Buddhist mandala.

action for the service of God and others. This has great implications in a patient's recovery.

Charity, the most genuine act of perfect love covers a multitude of sins. If we refuse or neglect to perform acts of love with our indifference, they will in turn form into human transgressions, negatively affecting souls and individual karma. Having a good heart with everyone, especially those who have transgressed against us, covers a multitude of sins or transgressions.

Another great virtue that covers a multitude of transgressions is humility. In order to grow without domineering, produce without possessing, and to do without presuming, one must lack pretension in one's life. Human life must be set with clear goals and objectives without the cloud of pretentiousness fogging it. When one lets go of the "*I*" and "*Mine*", of all pretensions, it will be easier to see and feel the "*We*" and the "*Ours*" in our lives.

Lastly, spiritual healing involves a whole new attitude, one with greater *depth and meaning* than the current one. It means going beyond the reality we have come to understand, to seeing a true cosmic existence and kinship with greater purpose, ultimately grasping the greater picture of life.

Such is the experience of a patient whose story will serve as testimony to the miracles that can occur here. At the age of 29, Matthew Ireland of Guilford, Vermont was diagnosed with a Stage IV inoperable brain tumor. After two years of conventional medical treatment with radiation and chemotherapy, the medical establishment could offer him no hope and following a neighbors advise to visit the Casa de Dom Inácio he turned to medium João de Deus for a possible healing. He was told to sit in current, so he did, for the following months. In his interview with Matt Goulding of Mens Health Magazine, Matthew comments: "I wasn't even a spiritual guy, I stayed because I had nothing to lose" (Goulding, 2007).

After his date with death had come and gone, Matthew returned to the states where he had a follow up MRI. His tumor had shrunk! His family and friends got him on the first flight back. This time he went straight to the current room, where he'd meditate for hours at a time. One day while he was in deep meditation, he felt a hand on his head. He opened his eyes to find John of God standing in front of him. "You are cured he said." João then instructed Matthew to go to the hospital and have tests done. Matthew immediately followed-up with an MRI just as João-in - entity had ordered. He presented himself at a large hospital in Goiania and had what would soon become his final MRI. The brain tumor was gone! All that was left was a bit of scar tissue. Matthew was given all the proof he needs, his life!!! What else could he ask for?

In another interview, John Quiñones (ABC correspondent who visited the casa in 2005 and had interviewed Matthew) consulted Dr. Oz for a second opinion regarding the remarkable improvement in Matthew's case. The doctor recognized Matthew had received effective medical intervention at the casa, "something stopped a process that normally is very aggressive" (Is John of God, 2005). He questioned if it had been something in the clinic's environment that may have contributed to his healing. Furthermore Dr. Oz added "I want to have the kind of music that gets him to meditate, the kind of biofeedback training and meditative training that will allow him to do what he needs to do to turn on his own body's healing mechanism." "That may be the greatest lesson of all here" (Is John of God, 2007). I must agree with Dr. Oz.

Matthew's story is without a doubt one of a miracle that occurred through God's infinite grace. In the following story God's grace too was accorded to a Brazilian woman who also received another healing miracle.

At the age of 38, Tania Maria Afonso, a devout catholic who ten years prior, had discovered the Kardecist teachings through the works of medium Chico Xavier, experienced an automobile accident that would forever change her life. Prior to losing control of her car, she heard a loud voice, warning her to slow down. The voice told her she was about to have an accident, and would suffer minor bruises but would survive. Tania had only sufficient time to reduce her car's speed to about 150 km/hr, and seconds later the front tire exploded. She was worried about hitting another car and killing or maiming innocent people.

She invoked the protection of God and all His angels. In an attempt to divert a collision with a nearby hill, she plunged her car into a small river.

When her car came to a stop she felt her seat belt pull and her spinal column tear in half, down the middle. She thought, if I'm dead why am I in so much pain? She opened the door to her car, she felt the water above her knees, and then realized she was still alive. She tried to locate her mobile phone, then turned to God to plead His help. She could hear the cars going by the road above her, but no one could see her. Comforted by the sweet fragrance of flowers she prayed and waited patiently. Forty minutes later two men rescued her. After one of the men shared with her that it was a voice that directed them to her.

They were approximately five kilometers away, when a voice told one of the men to turn back, to rescue a woman who was in the river in distress and in need of help. They turned back but saw nothing. But the voice insisted. They turned back again and looked below a bridge, but did not find her. Upon the persistence of the voice they turned back again and found her shortly after. She will remain forever grateful to the persistent good spirit and to the men's rescue efforts.

Tania was taken to a large metropolitan hospital in Goiania, in the state of Goiás, where she was admitted. The doctors found that she had an acute burst fracture of the T12 vertebral body (basically an explosion), with fractures on T10 and T11. That night while in the hospital, she received a visit from the benevolent spirit of Dr. Adolfo Bezerra de Menezes, who helped her with spiritual surgeries through the night, placing a spiritual device in her vertebrae, and told her she would eventually walk out of the hospital with her own strength and her own legs. The next morning Tania underwent surgical intervention, which the doctors warned: may result in her never walking again. They gave her a 2% chance of her ever recuperating her mobility to walk. To the amazement of her doctors, five days later she left the hospital walking with the help of crutches, but with her own two legs, as Dr Adolfo Bezerra de Menezes had advised her.

Her recovery continued well for the following three months, she almost got to the point where she would no longer need the help of the crutches she had been using. Then one day, she suffered a fall on a stairway, which set her back with greater pain and suffering. Her doctors told her the plate and pins they had inserted had moved with the fall, and would require a new surgery to put them back in place. At the time her physician also found two herniated discs. The problem now was that Tania had to raise a substantial amount of money to follow through with the surgery, which neither she nor her family, were prepared for. She had to seek medical help from a government hospital. But the wait was long.

Tania endured great pain, and had to stay in bed most of the time. Three months followed. Then one night as she laid in bed when a fair skinned man with light blue eyes appeared before her and told her "do not be afraid, I have come to help you." He came to her on several occasions and would bring her a vision of a beautiful place with lush and tranquil gardens and landscapes. The place had white and blue walls, and many people there spoke different languages and wore white clothing. She thought this hospital was in another country, and asked God how she was supposed to get there without the financial resources. No matter what, she trusted God. God knew what He was doing. She trusted He would take care of the details.

Tania would share her visions of this hospital with friends. Then one day, one of her mother's neighbors was sharing a story with them of a niece who was on her deathbed, and who after seeing famous healing medium João de Deus she miraculously recovered. The neighbor's niece now lived in Abadiania, approximately three and a half hours away from where Tania lived. Tania also learned that many foreigners frequented the Casa de Dom Inácio. Her mother reminded her of the visions she had of people speaking many different languages, suggesting, maybe this was the place she was supposed to go for healing. A month later Tania's uncle took her to the blessed spiritual hospital in Abadiania.

There, Tania stayed with the neighbor's niece for fifteen days. Upon her first visit before the entity, Dr. Valdivino told her he was waiting for her. Her cure would come through her work at the casa as a medium. He asked her to sit in the current room. In the current room, while Tania was in deep meditation she felt movement in her spinal column. She would see a bright green liquid penetrating her column. For the next 6 months she stayed with her new family of friends, in Abadiania, while serving at the casa and receiving spiritual treatment. She would still have to use her crutches, which she would only break away from, for showering and sleeping. She was told by the entity that when the bright green liquid color turned gold she would no longer need the crutches. Two weeks following the advise she had been given, an American friend she met through mutual friends, told her he saw a ball of gold light going in her direction. The next day, while she sat in current she saw the golden liquid being applied to her during meditation. This continued every day for the next week. Then the following week on June 24th, the feast day of St John the Baptist as well as the feast day of medium João, she felt she no longer needed the crutches that had supported her for all those months. She was so ecstatic; she danced!!! What Dr. Valdivino had told her was true. Her work as a medium would bring her cure. She was eternally grateful to God, to Christ, to the entities, to medium João, for helping her fully regain her health. She would remain forever humble, and she would continue to pray for all suffering souls, especially those who suffered more than she did. She prayed that their pain be lessened, that their ailments be replaced with complete health. She was happy to serve her Lord, and her Christ. One day the entities advised her she was being prepared to assist medium João and that eventually she would be ready to serve Jesus in other lands. She began to assist the entities and the medium with their healing works.

In December 2005 she met and fell in love with an American, Greg Stewart, and today she resides with him in Sacramento, California. Tania continues to do her work for all suffering souls. She wants everyone to know: "I wish at this time to express my eternal gratitude to my Lord, my Jesus, and to the untiring good spirits of Christ whom work with great love to bring peace and light to all suffering souls .... Believe, beloved brothers and sisters that read these blessed pages brought to our understanding by my beloved sister, that the love of God is everywhere, that we are His true children, and that He loves us unconditionally and eternally. Please understand that from the moment that we cease the battle against God's love and we allow His will in our lives, living a day at a time, loving one another, accepting and respecting each other just as we are with all of our imperfections and our individual qualities, that we shall all live a better and happier life because this is the only way we will learn to love, accept and respect all of humanity just as it is, with all it's imperfections and all of it's virtues. "

12

SPIRITUAL SURGERIES

Spiritual (*invisible* and *visible*) operations are quite common procedures in Brazil. Spiritual surgery, both *visible* and *invisible* (also referred to as: psychic surgery, trance surgery, and astral surgery) has become one of the most interesting and controversial types of healing procedures. Psychic surgery refers to a non-physical therapeutic technique that removes deep-rooted negative and stagnant energy that is almost always the root cause of many diseases in the physical body. It can also potentially remove or regenerate pathological matter. Psychic surgery in Brazil is somewhat different from the psychic surgeries conducted in the Phillipines, where incisions are done with bare hands. In Brazil *invisible* (psychic) spiritual surgery involves surgery that is done *without* the medium ever physically touching the person. It is done with the application of spiritual passes with the final objective of harmonizing the patient's ill energy.

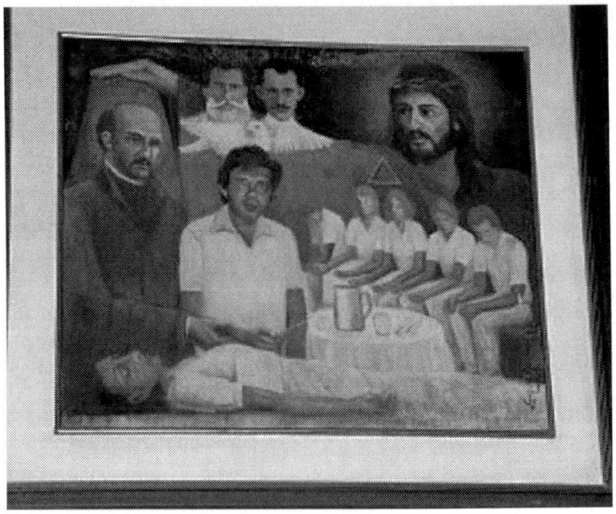

João, Christ, and entities doing spiritual surgery on a patient

A spiritual pass, as explained by Edgard Armond, in his book *Passes e Radiaçoes* (1950), is a non-material emanation of hand movements conducted by disincarnate spirits working through a medium, and directly affecting the patient's perispirit. Coming from superior spirits, the fluids that are transmitted to a healer during a spiritual pass, have greater healing power than those transmitted during magnetic passes (which involve no help from a spirit being, are done entirely by a living physical being). While the spiritual pass is magnetic in nature, it is believed that the quality of the fluid that is transmitted is definitely more invigorating than those transmitted during magnetic passes. Furthermore, magnetic passes address physical ailments with a physical remedy, by first removing negative energy from the physical body, but spiritual passes address spiritual ailments requiring spiritual healing.

In asking where the healing energy comes from, Brazilian spiritists believe it is energy that is all around us, in nature, in the cosmos. It is available for everyone to use for the greatest good. Gifted healing mediums have learned to tap into this energy and pass it on with the help of benevolent spirit beings

In both *invisible* and *visible* surgery, the medium's affected energy enters the patient's energy system (the auric field), and body to perform surgery, reaching the affected bodily organs and systems. It is important that no one apart from the healer and patient use up the auric space between the two.

With *invisible* spiritual surgery, a surgery is done without the use of any physical surgical instruments, as there is no need for physical incision. As is the case at the casa de Dom Inacio, all patients needing an *invisible* spiritual surgery can be accommodated within the same physical space (room) and within one time period. João in entity walks around the room blessing and healing everyone in the name of Christ while everyone, sitting in current is in deep meditation. Furthermore, instruments that are used in invisible spiritual surgery do not have the physical density that would allow a person with normal sense to see or feel them. Nonetheless, patients have reported movement within the auric field and manipulation of material under the skin while undergoing a spiritual surgical intervention.

In both *visible* and *invisible* spiritual surgeries, it is believed that radiant fluids interpenetrate the healer's spiritual body. The healer then transmits these fluids to the auric field, skin, tissue or organ of the patient and subsequently once they reach the cellular life field, they bombard the atoms, elevate their intimate vibration and give cells a more intense vitality. The healer with the help of spirit entities extirpates diseased growths, regenerates atrophies, unties obstructed circulation, reduces stenosis (an abnormal condition characterized by the constriction of an opening or passageway), and regenerates irreparable organs.

"The healer then transmits these fluids to the auric field, skin, tissue or organ of the patient and subsequently once they reach the cellular life field, they bombard the atoms, elevate their intimate vibration and give cells a more intense vitality."

By treating the patient's *perispirit*, the medium alters the patient's disturbed constitution, reestablishing the patient's natural organization. This realigning of the *perispirit* with the physical body reestablishes the necessary harmony for the patient's recovery, thus explaining spiritual passes and surgeries as the Natural Law of Equilibrium taking place during the exchange of essential bodily fluids. During the contact between the healing medium and patient, the medium positions himself in such a way that allows the universe to vibrate in harmony with him and his patient. Healing energy must flow from the cosmos to the benevolent spirit, to the healer, to the patient, with love, compassion and trust in the Creator.

Once a *visible* or *invisible* spiritual surgery is complete, and a particular organ or tissue has been regenerated or excised the medium directly sends healing energy to the specific area to recompose the affected organ or tissue. In doing so, he reestablishes its function. The spirit entities channel spiritual energies and principles to support the patient's own internal healing process. This is how healing is achieved, the function of the organ is recuperated, and the patient's aspect of the disease is modified.

João de Deus' primary method of healing in his earlier years, were physical surgeries (*visible*, on-the-flesh). He continues to do a limited amount of these surgeries only because he believes they serve the function of strengthening people's faith in his work. João's physical (*visible*) surgeries are performed in front of an entire patient group that is present at the casa. The patients, whom João-in-entity operates (*visibly*), stand before the audience with their eyes closed, and are being operated during meditation while the spirits direct the healers hands where healing is needed. Physical (*visible*) surgeries are performed on those who volunteer, must be 18 to 52 years old, and must not have been recently subjected to radiation or chemotherapy. The latter patient groups whom cannot opt for a *visible* surgery will be offered *invisible* spiritual surgery, which provides the same results. So long as the spirit entity is in agreement, those who volunteer for *visible* spiritual surgery (since spirit entities do not always approve a patient request) will receive one. The method (*visible* or *invisible* [physical or spiritual] intervention) that is chosen for the patient depends on what is best for him, and lies at the discretion of João in entity.

Most of the visible spiritual surgeries performed by medium João in entity involve either 1) inserting forceps into the patient's nasal cavity followed with turning and twisting, 2) scraping the cornea with what appears to be a small kitchen knife, or 3) cutting the flesh to remove pathological matter. The first two procedures are said to have deeper therapeutic significance. The first is said to stimulate the pituitary glands, as well as the endocrine glands.

These *visible* and *invisible* surgeries have shown pain is absent in most cases, despite the lack of (chemically) sterile procedures and anesthesia – although "astral" anesthesia and antiseptics are used. The "spirit anesthesia" allows a patient to stand while

"The spirit entities channel spiritual energies and principles to support the patient's own internal healing process. This is how healing is achieved, the function of the organ is recuperated, and the patient's aspect of the disease is modified."

undergoing the surgical intervention, and has shown patients to talk clearly when they are asked a question, signaling an active consciousness on behalf of the patient. With those surgeries involving physical (*visible*) spiritual surgery, very little bleeding from the physical incisions or removal of tissue has been documented thus demonstrating they are a most unique, and non-invasive, form of surgery.

Although *visible* surgeries at the casa are still done, João and the entities perform more *invisible* (astral/psychic) surgeries. Patients who have undergone *invisible* as well as *visible* surgeries report post-surgical symptoms for the following weeks. Post surgical instructions are to be followed just as would be expected with allopathic surgical procedures, which will include limited physical activity, refraining from sexual activity for forty days, etc. There is a mandatory 24-hour recovery period immediately following an operation. Whenever possible, one is not to move far from the *pousada* or hotel room. In both *visible* and *invisible* surgery cases, x-rays have been performed following spiritual surgeries, and have revealed sutures had been placed, indicating a surgically spiritual (*visible* or *invisible*) intervention had taken place.

Spiritual surgery and healing can perhaps be best understood within the context of natural laws and principles. No matter what type of disease is present, it is believed that it possesses an energetic root that becomes lodged in or around a particular organ, in one of the chakras, or in the aura. This semi-material mechanism is essential to the understanding of *visible* and *invisible* spiritual surgical interventions.

Traditional surgical procedures remove the "blocked energy" at the *physical* level – the tissue, organs, or any other type of physical anomaly generated by the process of disease. Physical surgery only addresses the physical area of the body. On the other hand, both *visible* and *invisible* spiritual surgery act directly upon the *root* of the problem, the primary *cause* of the problem. The spiritual surgical removal of blocked energy (which is done in both *visible* and *invisible* surgery) is processed in a painless manner, without physically cutting (in *invisible* spiritual surgery), without anesthesia, without any risks, or possibility of any damage.

"Physical surgery only addresses the physical area of the body. On the other hand, both visible and invisible spiritual surgery, act directly upon the root of the problem, the primary cause of the problem."

Traditional medical surgery is significant within the sphere of the physical body and spiritual surgery (unlike traditional surgery), performs beyond that conventional therapeutic (physical) arena – reaching the "energetic organs," chakras, "bioplasmic body," and the aura, [done by removing blocked energy, negative feelings, "*miasmas energéticas*" (a type of psychic parasite that has been formed by heavy and dense energy)] – areas not addressed by conventional therapies and require a transcendental approach to understand them in their entirety. Therefore, healing can be seen as an attunement to Divine love and energy that a healing medium passes on to his patients to rebalance their own physical, emotional, and spiritual energies, something allopathic doctors are not trained to do.

It is important to note here that while the U.S. Federal Trade Commission declared psychic surgery to be nothing but a total hoax, fakery and fraud in 1975, then again in 1990 the American Cancer Society cautioned against it, many ill patients continue to seek spiritual healers and healing mediums. And while there are individuals who seek their care, there are those who have dedicated their entire life to bringing down *all* psychic healers. While there are those who are illegitimate, there also exist those who are equally legitimate. The work of a skeptic as well as academia is nonetheless needed to help society identify the fraudulent ones. But this is to say not all mediumistic healers are quacks.

Patients may not necessarily understand the concepts of mediumistic medicine, but imagining their illnesses may have been caused by a shift in their spiritual axis, may help shield them from the glaring light of scientific reality. They may find themselves believing when others they come to know share with them a true story of hope. This can help ward off despair and thus may help promote healing.

The idea that human beings are composed of energy fields and that a person's energy can be "balanced" or "decongested" is revolutionary. If and when proven true, it would overthrow the paradigm that has governed medical science for over a century. Some individuals are beginning to acknowledge scientific studies do not need to be statistically significant to prove or disprove anything. For these individuals, hope and the will of the Creator are what really matter.

To obtain further information about spiritual surgeries and the work that goes on at the Casa de Dom Inácio please refer to the useful casa (house) rules at: www.johnofgod.com/casaguide.pdf. If you are planning a trip It is also recommended to check John of God's traveling schedule at www.friendsofthecasa.org to assure he will be at the casa during the time you are planning to visit. For your information there are many casa guides whom coordinate trips to this healing sanctuary several times a year. Both authors Josie RavenWing, and Mr. Estrich-Pellegrino as well as many others, provide their service as guides to the casa. Their website information is listed in the bibliographic section of this book. Be advised you will need a valid passport and a current Brazilian visa to enter Brazil.

PART FOUR

CHANGING THE MODEL TO INCLUDE MORAL AND SOCIAL HEALTH

13

HUMANISTIC MEDICINE INVOLVES AN INTEGRATIVE APPROACH: WHY OUTDATED MODELS MUST CHANGE

Our current classic healthcare system unfortunately is still modeled on disease patterns that were predominant in the first half of the 20th century. From treating acute conditions beginning with the epidemics of the latter half of the 19th century, to trauma and infectious diseases in the first half of the 20th century, to treating chronic illness from 1950 to the present, the healthcare model has evolved without ever modifying it's therapeutic interventions.

A system originally designed to treat acute, short-term and individual episodes of illness that was discontinuous in nature, was also used to treat chronic illness (characterized as long-term and continuous) as if it too, were a series of acute and separate episodes. If chronic illness is and will continue to be the prevalent health problem, the current model, no longer suitable, demands attention and modification.

Chronic illness often beginning early in life, long before overt symptoms appear and before medical treatment is directed toward them, allows disease to become firmly implanted long before symptoms call attention. Unlike acute conditions, chronic illness once present, usually remains with the patient forever, meaning that the classic model of medicine does not include treatment modalities aimed at completely healing the disease, and instead treats only it's more prominent symptoms or external manifestations.

Short intensive interventions that may have effectively treated acute illness episodes have not been able to provide appropriate or effective treatment modalities for chronic illness. The case for cancer in the United States demonstrates cancer survival rates after diagnosis, have made slight improvement in the past few years. Despite the vast medical and pharmaceutical interventions, and tremendous financial resources directed to research and treatment interventions they have not significantly improved incidence rates. As reported in the Annual Report to the Nation on the Status of Cancer, 1975-2004: "Overall cancer death rates decreased by 2.1% per year from 2002–2004, but the incidence rate was *higher* for stomach, liver, cervix, kidney, and gallbladder" (SEER, 2007). The prospect for the future is bleak, if nothing is *fundamentally* changed within the current paradigm.

Obviously, when an entirely different set of health conditions arose these required an entirely different array of services and interventions to ensure a healthcare system that would be appropriate and responsive to the changing health problems of the times. When this did not occur, it created increased frustration compounded by the complexity, bureaucracy, and escalating expenses exacerbated by a growing number of increasing morbidity and mortality rates, as is evident in our current overall health crisis.

A report of the World Health Organization (WHO) claims the top ten leading causes of death in the United States are 1) ischaemic heart disease 2) cerebrovascular disease 3) lung cancers 4) chronic obstructive pulmonary disease 5) alzheimer and other dementias 6) diabetes mellitis 7) colon and rectum cancers 8) lower respiratory infections 9) breast cancer, and 10) road traffic accidents (WHOSIS, US, 2002). Cancer for the US ranked thrice among the top ten list (lung, colon, and breast cancers respectively), while cancer did not make Brazil's top ten leading causes of death for the same year (WHOSIS, Brazil, 2002).

The deaths reported by Brazil that were related to neuropsychiatric conditions were also less prevalent than those reported by the US. Brazil reported 23,829 deaths in 2002 (or a rate of 13 per 100,000 persons) while the US reported 154,290 (or 53 per 100,000 persons) (WHO Global InfoBase). A significant difference in the number of deaths by neuropsychiatric conditions could reflect the holistic approach Brazilian Spiritists have adopted in dealing with mental health treatment.

There are important repercussions, as they are evident in our nation's overall health. A report published in the Journal of the American Medical Association (JAMA), titled *Is US Health Really the Best in the World?* (2000), written by Dr. Barbara Starfield, of the John Hopkins School of Hygiene and Public Health, shows that medical errors may be the third leading cause of death in the United States. This type of red alert, pointing to the imperfections of our current health system, should encourage classic medicine to identify the need for fundamental change and to look at other paradigms that offer more effective, and less costly outcomes.

In comparing Brazil's mortality rates to the US, specifically deaths caused by malignant neoplasms, the following observation is made from the reports of the World Health Organization (WHO). The Deaths caused by malignant neoplasms, last reported for 2002, the United States reported 558,643. The death rate per 100,000 individuals was 191. Brazil reported 177,748 deaths caused by malignant neoplasms, with a rate of 100 per 100,000 individuals. While the amount of money the US expended on health, (per capita), was 3 times more than the amount spent by Brazil (per capita). The United States spent 6,096.00 per capita, while Brazil spent only 1520.00. When .19% of the American population die from malignant neoplasms, vs. only .1% of the Brazilian population we find a rather *concerning* difference in mortality rates, .18% to be more precise. Keeping in mind that the US spends three times more money on the resources directed to reduce the number of deaths related to cancer, the results are calling for fundamental change in the way treatment is directed (WHO Global InfoBase, Deaths Caused By Malignant Neoplasms, 2002).

Unlike acute conditions that can be healed with one or few treatment interventions, chronic illness requires long-term treatment, and optimal *prevention* methods; conducive only to a healthcare system that is in itself long-term, continuous, and preventative in nature. A model that would address social health and include a stronger preventative focus would help bring major changes to an individual's knowledge of disease, personal values, and behavioral norms.

As noted by Dr. James Hospedales, chief of the Unit of Chronic Disease of the Pan American Health Organization (PAHO), it is not only the health sector that needs to be involved, but the active participation of education, trade and agriculture, finance, and planning sectors along with the private sector, communications media, food companies, and civil society, are all being called to answer this global health crisis of growing chronic illness (Epstein, 2007).

While there have been changes in healthcare organization (from traditional healthcare to managed care), these changes have had some ameliorating effect on the administrative organizational aspect of healthcare management, but have not shown significant improvement in the effectiveness of treatment interventions, despite the great advances in technology. Aside from the organizational structure of the healthcare system (that has somewhat improved its efficiency in the fiscal, organizational, and utilization areas of healthcare) it is the treatment interventions that are calling for a much needed review.

Extending re-organizational parameters should begin with 1) a careful revision of both the current code of ethics, and 2) healthcare policy development that is not shaped by major economic market and political factors. To bring back the sacredness originally intended in medicine, a closer look at what medical schools are teaching future generations of health practitioners is also needed. Training that would involve healing the entire organism, rather than only pacifying ill physical symptoms or relieving pain temporarily, would more suitably serve a patient's needs.

For this to occur institutions of higher learning, particularly medical schools, will need to request from their students more receptivity to new approaches that look at a patient in a holistic form, as an individual connected (or disconnected) from the universal life current. Looking at patients with a unique set of conditions and ill symptoms, and implementing individualized treatment plans for them, rather than categorizing them with standard diagnosis and prognosis protocols, and a generalized treatment plan, would again, serve the patient's needs more adequately.

Beginning with treatment modalities that have been developed to plug a patient into an established conventional theoretical orientation, rather than to design a treatment modality that will suit the *individual* patient needs. By superficially treating a diseased body, unhealthy toxic waste affecting mental and physical health, can develop into a major health threat.

As healing practitioners, doctors should be able to instill confidence, faith, and hope in their patients; something institutions of higher learning, and present healthcare system, do not address.

The spiritual body, particularly the patient's mental and emotional condition (containing memories of one's former lives), cannot be completely addressed or resolved by maintenance-oriented care, a drug prescription regimen that only suppresses symptoms, and/or conventional psychotherapy which is limited to a traditional patient's medical history. Since medication, conventional medical treatments and surgeries, electro-convulsive therapy, and conventional psychotherapy may not completely address this aspect of the patient's health problem, healing mediums, Spiritual-Medical specialists who can provide transcendental therapeutic intervention, are best prepared for this unique and specialized task.

Brazilian healing mediums and *casas* are continuously calling attention from traditional healthcare practitioners, scientists, and mental health professionals because it is through the Spirit of truth and knowledge that they are gaining an integral understanding of health and illness. A patient's evolutionary biography, which in medical terms comprises a most comprehensive patient medical history, is helping conventional practitioners understand that the key to healing a patient's ill biological composition lies beyond the traditionally limited patient medical history.

To better read, interpret, diagnose, and treat disease, physicians require a humbling approach to their noble profession, as has been the expressed by Dr. Uehara, a medico-espirita of cardiovascular specialty from Sao Paulo, Brazil. He has been attending the Casa de Dom Inácio, and assisting medium João for over ten years. He believes all western trained physicians need to acknowledge medicine as belonging to the superior realms. For this to happen, he says, "doctors need to humble themselves to the Creator." This is why he has chosen to serve at the casa, traveling from Sao Paulo to Abadiania, numerous times a year. It serves to remind him of his humble position.

Scientific progress in the seventeenth century, proceeding directly from an empirical standpoint, had to discard important long-held theological (moral) and philosophical orientations from the book of nature. While scientific progress improved research techniques, and advanced technology to impressive heights, it had deleterious effects that transformed important moral values and consequently affected political, economic, and social structures.

The secularization of a new era began more than four centuries ago and the ill effects and conditions continue to be felt today. To revert to the original sacredness of human life will require a return to the dualistic, transcendental system that will permit symbolic and mystical to go hand in hand with the empirical and practical.

Religion and Science being the two levers of human intelligence, and coming from the same divine source, can only lead to the One source, and cannot contradict each other, as it would be inconsistent with divine design.

The root of the misconception thus lies only in the resulting incomplete and limited one-sided views each hold of each other, deriving from a most profound conception of *Truth* (*that which is considered to be the supreme reality and to have the ultimate meaning and value of existence; conforming to knowledge, fact, or logic)*. Truth will be achieved when both scientific and religious levers have been equally activated.

The time has arrived for science and religion to complement each other. "Science must see beyond matter and acknowledge a spiritual perspective, religion must stop ignoring the fundamental laws of matter. Only in this way will both sides come together and learn to lean on each other" (Kardec, 2000, p. 33).

"The missing link is contained in the knowledge of the laws that govern the non-physical (spiritual) realm and its interactions with the world of matter – laws, it should be pointed out, as constant as the ones that govern the movement of the stars and the existence of living beings. Once these interactions are empirically demonstrated, we will see things in a new light. Faith will speak to reason; reason will find nothing illogical in faith, materialism will be overcome" (Kardec, 2000, p 33).

14

BUILDING NEW HEALTH PARTNERSHIPS WHILE IMPROVING SOCIAL CONDITIONS: *TRABALHANDO*

Brazilian spiritist-doctors use the same therapies allopathic doctors learned in medical school, but further to the biomedical medicines and surgeries, Spiritist-doctors have also come to rely on homeopathy, acupuncture, trans-personal psychology, memory regression therapies, and spiritist complementary therapy (involving mediumistic healers). These spiritist-doctors believe that the materialistic classic paradigm is in its final stages of "exhaustion" and is depending on the future generation of academics they produce to reshape medicine.

Preparing for the future requires an expansive vision that will enable the humanistic and transcendental medical model of the future to be characterized by a wide-ranging representation of healing traditions, faiths, nationalities, ethnic and traditional points-of-view; a vision that demands a delicate look at the web of life in its entirety.

"These medical-spiritist doctors believe that the materialistic classic paradigm is in its final stages of "exhaustion" and is depending on the future generation of academics they produce to reshape medicine."

Just as the scientific arena in its evolutionary discourse has shared among the various scientific disciplines it's methods, statistical information, and results that have contributed to it's advancement, an integrative model of health for the entire human race will require the medical community transcend borders (as Brazilians are now doing) that reach out to the international community.

The invaluable cooperation of other world spiritual and healing wisdom offers the medical community a new constellation of conceptions, values, perceptions and practices that may assist them in forming a new model that will not only improve individual physical health but also improve overall global moral, mental, and social health. Fostering universal mental, moral, and social health, as many Brazilians have come to engage in, is achieved through charitable works done in collaboration of the common good, what they refer to as "*trabalhar.*"

Trabalhar is an important edifying concept to master in one's lifetime, preferably early on. It is the accumulation of good karma one accrues; it is the only ticket to one's salvation. So the younger one is to acknowledge and comprehend this Law, the greater the amount of good karma one can accrue and take to the afterlife; the higher one will ascend.

Alone the non-cyclical concept of nature and human life that has existed throughout the last 2000 years throughout most of the world, or at least in the New World, when presented in its new light of repetitive cycles of death and rebirth, can bring a new and powerful meaning to the lives of many.

Understanding Natural Law's *cyclical* nature (that beings die and are born again to balance karma with good deeds); understanding that all things pass (as seasons will always come again), that life is impermanent (physical existence always ends), should help individuals better cope with the realities of pain, suffering, and death.

Fearing the loss of life (what is seen as the *only* human existence), or fear of death, undoubtedly delays human spiritual growth. By not conquering the spiritual strength that is required to achieve inner peace, and serenity that will help maintain a state of equilibrium in the circles of human struggle, evolutionary progress could be difficult to obtain.

> *"Society could gain inner peace in knowing physical life is impermanent, but spiritual life is eternal."*

Only when humanity embraces a new perspective, a true perspective of *the cyclical nature of all things*, will the spirit gain a wider vision, an expansion of consciousness, a communal mindset that allies itself with cooperation, collaboration and collectiveness. Society could gain inner peace in knowing physical life is impermanent, but spiritual life is eternal. In short, humanity should be a more harmonious and productive people.

Having the potential to create more socially responsible individuals, by positively affecting many of society's ills and having the capability to reduce abusive and suicidal tendencies, urban violence, and to increase harmony in an individual's life – are all progressive in nature.

In incorporating diagnostic and treatment modalities from all of the world's spiritual and healing traditions, the model of integral health offers a *universal code of human ethics* in the practice of humanistic and integrative medicine. Important contributions from the world's major spiritual and healing traditions used in this new treatment repertoire, is providing Brazilian Spiritists essential guidelines required for ethical living in both private and public life.

Undeniably, this integrative model of health offers a unique "unifying" aspect to the healing experience. In recognizing all religious belief-systems actually descend from the same "one-ness" of the divine source, patients are finding themselves reconnecting with a *common* higher self.

Sharing similar ill physical or spiritual conditions, patients are able to follow a universal healing approach and are being reawakened to a new spiritual reality, one that takes on a new dimension. Healing occurs while removing walls that previously were the boundaries to separatism, stereotypes, and misunderstandings that had led many to much of their unhappiness.

Mediumistic, humanistic, or transcendental medicine, however one prefers to term it, will help individuals recognize the importance of moral health in the context of complete health; requiring a multidisciplinary cooperation between *spiritual science* and *classical science*. By patients educating themselves with both spiritual and material knowledge, they can grow to be more discerned individuals, and thus learn to transform irrational situations into reasonable ones. By morally educating the soul, patients can reach higher levels of consciousness that could allow them to self-integrate back into the sacred web of life.

While there are many definite health benefits to

be gained from adapting the dualistic Brazilian model of health, not all would embrace it. Unfortunately at this time, transplanting mediumistic medicine to the U.S. would pose a major legal challenge. Perhaps after the relatively young field of parapsychology gains stronger academic and scientific support, and validation (particularly mediumistic healing), it could influence a new perspective on the scientific, medical, and legal arenas that at this time will not allow it to flourish. Not until it is fully accepted and accredited will it be permitted to coexist with classical medicine. In the meantime, there is much that can still be done to improve the current health crisis.

> *"Only when humanity embraces a new perspective, a true perspective of the cyclical nature of all things, will the spirit gain a wider vision, an expansion of consciousness, a communal mindset that allies itself with cooperation, collaboration and collectiveness."*

To begin, classic medicine can admit the current model is outdated and requires major modification. This alone is a start. Recognizing the importance of preventative-oriented care, and adding much needed emphasis on the importance of patient education. Biomedicine would also benefit from acknowledging important contributions coming from all healing and spiritual traditions and therapies. These could have definite implications in the healing process.

The concept of *casas* as healing sanctuaries is extremely important to replicate here as it has proven success that would likely also replicate anywhere outside of Brazil. Establishing healthcare facilities that serve the same purpose, to educate, spiritually guide, and heal both the spiritual and physical ailments of a patient, offers great potential in reducing mental illness and in significantly changing current morbidity and mortality rates.

The setting would reflect that of a healing sanctuary, with plenty of space allocated for meditation rooms, which would serve as current rooms. As in *casas*, these rooms provide a place to meditate, to harness and redirect healing energy. Qualified energy healers from various world-healing traditions could assist patients with realigning and rebalancing their damaged or weakened energy systems.

As a healing sanctuary the grounds would also reflect a peaceful and most serene landscape, surrounded with waterfalls, abundant and lush gardens, and awe-inspiring sacred art from the different world spiritual traditions located throughout the casa walls, making it a most sacred space, accessible to all.

The volunteer medical staff would coexist with naturopathic doctors, spiritual healers from the different traditions, energy healers, and spiritual representatives (e.g. rabbi's, priests, ministers, etc) on the premises to help those who have forgotten basic human principles and require a mentor or specialist that works with them in surrendering their will to God. In preparing them to serve selflessly so they may receive both successes and failures with equal calmness as granted by their Creator.

These health facilities would also serve as research centers that would bring a collaborative working environment permitting many different world healing and spiritual traditions to come together. Multidisciplinary efforts joined to provide a more integrative solution to the current global health crisis should offer an exchange of valuable medical research, and literature for researchers as well as for patients and the general public.

The ultimate goal in replicating the concept of *casas* in the United States would be to produce as many "live antennas" by preparing souls in the direction of heaven.

15

FINAL THOUGHTS

Undoubtedly, Brazilian spiritual and psychic healing require an understanding of Brazilian culture, the particular way in which they view the world, their unique position in the general progress of humanity, and their passion for the continuous evolution of the world's soul. Brazilians, believing their land and people have been given the task of alleviating human suffering, humanizing medicine, and christianizing humanity, turn out to be light bearers in a project involving major world progress.

Not until all men cease to indulge in the vine of authority and personal ambition will Brazil's *medico-espiritas* (spiritist-doctors) and soul doctors (healing mediums) come close to their monumental goals – integral and transcendental medicine – one that exists in the absence of bureaucratic hierarchies, and inflated fees. When the objectives of medicine are no longer overshadowed by the interests of insurance companies, nor of the larger medical, economic, and political conglomerates, and instead are met with a most basic and practical application of the pedagogical Christian principles of spiritual and physical health, then medicine will achieve a greater level.

Working to create a better world where wisdom, faith, reason, and love, are *fully* integrated involves a *grand* effort. Important spiritual hearts and minds of the ancient world came to show humanity the way. Christ, as well as other enlightened minds, brought a greater and clearer understanding of the way. And the current humanistic health movement in Brazil will help humanity complete its transcendental and evolutionary project of integrative medicine.

Kardec, Bezerra de Menezes, Chico Xavier, João de Deus, Divaldo Franco, Suely Schubert, Brolio, Costa, Armand, Krippner, RavenWing, Estrich-Pellegrino, Dossey, Brennan, and Myss, as well as many other courageous souls (both carnate and disincarnate) whose names are not included here, not only understand invaluable spiritual and healing truths from the many world traditions, but also, are acting upon a most honorable oath to defend God's creation, even when their messages do not conform to the times.

If humanity had never allowed new revolutionary ideas to coexist with those of the paradigms of it's time, and had simply discarded the ideas because they were beyond the thinking parameters of the time, the evolutionary progress made in all areas, scientific, theological, and philosophical would have never been accomplished.

Each idea from all disciplines, whether scientific, philosophical, or theological, comprises the whole. "The fact that honorable and highly accomplished individuals, after extensive inquiry, have come forth in defense of the new ideas, makes those ideas at least a distinct possibility" (Kardec, 2002, p.19). Undoubtedly spiritual healing offers both, great spiritual value, and intellectual worth.

BRAZILIAN AND UNIVERSAL PRAYERS

PRAYER FOR INNER PEACE

Lord Almighty and All Powerful, ***Guard carefully***........

...My trust in You and in myself,
...My conscience, that it always be at peace,
...My time, occupying it in fruitful endeavors,
...My speech, that it always be constructive,
...My prayers, while working edifyingly,
...My hope, while serving others,
...My patience, while working for the common good,
...My opinion, that it never lack love,
...My blessing, of a greater understanding,
...My participation, with the progress of humanity,
...My attitude, that it never lack compassion,
...My truth, always illuminated with Your love,
...My recollection, of all my wrongdoings,
...My fidelity, of all my undertakings,
...My forgiving, that it always be unconditional,
...My devotion, to higher learning,
...My gesture, of sympathy,
...My smile, of encouragement,
...My spontaneous assistance to those in need,
...My simplicity, in all habits,
...My spirit, always renewed,
...My wisdom, of tolerance,
...My courage, to forget myself in the service of others,
...My perseverance, only of all that is good.

May I conserve such personal transformations, in my daily experiences, to acquire the science of inner peace with the privilege of finding happiness through my work, amidst the climate of love. Amen

MY DAILY OFFERING

I adore You my Lord, I Love You with all of my heart. I thank you for creating me, and for allowing me to know Christ, for having conserved my health and my life. I offer You my day: all of my actions, that they correspond with Your most holy will. That I may do everything for Thy honor and glory; for my peace, and the peace of the world. Free me from sin, danger, and evil. May Your grace, blessings, light, and presence always be with me and with all of my loved ones. Amen

ACT OF CONSECRATION TO THE HOLY SPIRIT

On my knees, before the great multitude of heavenly witnesses, I offer myself soul and body to You, Eternal Spirit of God.

I adore the brightness of Your purity, the unerring keenness of Your justice, and the might of Your love. You are the strength and light of my soul. In You I live and move and am. I desire never to grieve You by unfaithfulness to grace, and I pray with all of my heart to be kept from the smallest sin against You. Mercifully guard my every thought and grant that I may always watch for Your light and listen to Your voice and follow Your gracious inspirations. I cling to You and give myself to You and ask You, by Your compassion, to watch over me in my weakness. Holding the pierced feet of Jesus and looking at his five wounds and trusting in His precious blood and adoring His opened side and stricken heart, I implore You, adorable Spirit, helper of my infirmity, so to keep me in Your grace that I may never sin against You. Give me grace, O Holy Spirit, Spirit of the Father and the Son, to say to You always and everywhere, “Speak, Lord, for Your servant is listening.” Amen

PRAYER FOR THE SEVEN GIFTS OF THE HOLY SPIRIT

O Lord Jesus Christ, who before ascending into heaven promised to send the Holy Spirit to finish Your work in the souls of Your apostles and disciples, grant the same Holy Spirit to me that he may perfect in my soul the work of Your grace and Your love. Grant me the Spirit of Wisdom, that I may despise the perishable things of this world and aspire only after the things that are eternal; the Spirit of Understanding, to enlighten my mind with the light of Your divine truth; the Spirit of Counsel, that I may ever choose the surest way of pleasing God and gaining heaven, the Spirit of Fortitude, that I may bear my cross with You and that I may overcome with courage all the obstacles that oppose my salvation; the Spirit of Knowledge, that I may know God and know myself and grow perfect in the science of the saints; the Spirit of Piety, that I may find the service of God sweet and amiable; the Spirit of Love, that I may be filled with a loving reverence toward God and may dread in any way to displease Him.

Mark me, Dear Lord, with the sign of Your True Disciples and animate me in all things with Your Spirit. Amen

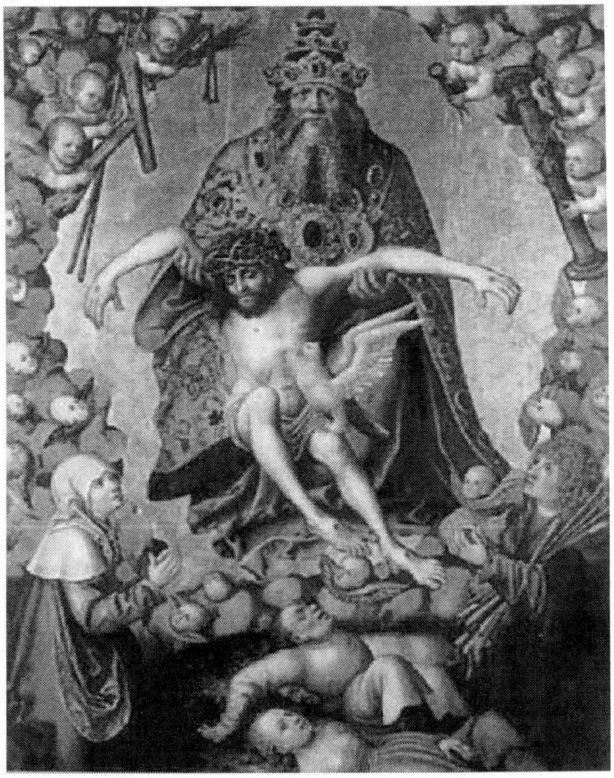

Our Lord Jesus Christ, who on the cross gave for us Your life: Of your opened side You have brought forth for the world a spring of Life, and resurrected You have given us Your peace and Your joy. Allow us the glance of true faith that we are able to astonish ourselves and welcome the love of God the Father whom You have manifested. Help us to live following your steps impelled by the Holy Spirit who you endowed to us the day of our baptism. Nurture us along our paths with your Body and Blood in the Eucharist. Teach us to love all as You have loved us. Fortify us, that we are able to take up our crosses and help take them to all of our brothers. Strengthen our hope until we share with you eternal life. Amen

PRAYER OF CARITAS

God, our Father, who is all power and goodness, please give strength to those who are experiencing pain and anguish. Give Light to those who seek the truth, and fill the human heart with love and compassion. God please give the travéler the star that guides, solace to those in pain, and rest to the sick and weary.

Father! Give the guilty repentance, the spirit, truth, give the child guidance, the orphan a father. Lord! Let Your goodness encompass everything that You have created. Clemency, my God, to those who do not know You. Hope to those who are in pain.

Let Your will allow the consoling spirits to spread peace, hope and faith everywhere. God! May a single ray of light, a spark of Your divine love, blaze the Earth. Let us drink from the fountain of that infinite and fruitful goodness and all tears will be dried and all pain lessened.

A single heart, a single thought will rise to You, like a cry of gratitude and love. Like Moses on the mountain, we await You with open arms, Oh Almighty! Oh Greatness! Oh All Powerful, Oh All Beauty! Oh All perfection! We wish in some way to receive your mercy.

God, give us the power to help everyone progress; that we may rise up to You. Give us pure charity, give us faith and reason, give us simplicity that will make our souls the mirror into which Your divine image may be reflected. Amen.

PRAYER TO ANGEL HAAMIAH

In the name of the Almighty Creator, whose truth is universal and absolute, I call upon you, great Angel Haamiah, with an honest and open heart to guide me in my quest for spiritual knowledge. May I know the true from the false, and may I not be misled by deceivers. I honor you and thank you for granting me your protection, as is your righteous duty. In the name of the Almighty. Amen

THE LORD'S PRAYER

(translated from ARAMAIC, the language spoken by Jesus)

O Birther! Father-Mother of the Cosmos,
Focus your light within us - make it useful:
Create your reign of unity now –
Your one desire then acts with ours,
As in all light, so in all forms.
Grant what we need each day in bread and insight.
Loose the cords of mistakes binding us,
As we release the strands we hold of others' guilt.
Don't let surface things delude us,
But free us from what holds us back.
From you is born all ruling will,
The power and the life to do,
The song that beautifies all,
From age to age it renews.

Truly - power to these statements – May they be the ground from which all my actions grow. Amen.

PRAYER TO OUR LADY OF THE ROSARY

O Virgin Mary, grant that the recitation of thy Rosary may be for me each day, in the midst of my manifold duties, a bond of unity in my actions, a tribute of filial piety, a sweet refreshment, an encouragement to walk joyfully along the path of duty. Grant, above all, O Virgin Mary, that the study of thy twenty mysteries may form in my soul, little by little, a luminous atmosphere – pure, strengthening, and fragrant – which may penetrate my understanding, my will, my heart, my memory, my imagination, my whole being.

Thus shall I acquire the habit of praying while I work, without the aid of formal prayers, by interior acts of admiration and of supplication, or by aspirations of love, I ask this of thee, O Queen of the Most Holy Rosary. Amen

(For those who are unfamiliar with the Holy Rosary you may go to: http://mostholyrosary.org/ for a blessed ROSARY experience).

PRAYER OF ST. DOMINIC

O holy priest of God and glorious patriarch, St. Dominic, thou who was the friend, the well-beloved son and confidant of the Queen of Heaven, and did work so many miracles by the power of the Holy Rosary, have regard for my necessities. On earth you opened your heart to the miseries of your fellow men and your hands were strong to help them; now in heaven your charity has not grown less nor has your power waned. Pray for me to the Mother of the Rosary and to her divine Son, for I have great confidence that through your assistance I shall obtain the favor I so much desire. Amen

SOUL OF CHRIST AND SOUL OF MARIA

Soul of Jesus and Soul of Maria, sanctify us. Heart of Jesus and Heart of Maria, save us. Blood of Jesus which is the blood of Maria, inebriate us. Water from the side of Christ and tears of Maria, wash us. Passion of Christ and sorrows of Maria, strengthen and comfort us. Within thy wounds and the wounds of your mother's trespassed heart, hide us. From the malignant one always defend us. At the hour of our death call us. And bid us to come to Thee, to place us next to Thee, so that now and forever, we may repeat incessantly: Holy, Holy, Holy, is our Lord all love and mercy and Holy, Holy, Holy, is Maria Mother of God and our Mother, universal mediator of all graces. Amen

THE GREAT INVOCATION

From the point of Light within the Mind of God
let Light stream forth into the minds of men.
Let Light descend on Earth.

From the point of Love within the Heart of God
Let love stream forth into the hearts of men.
May Christ return to Earth.

From the center where the Will of God is known
Let purpose guide the little wills of men –
The purpose, which the Masters know and serve.

From the center which we call the race of men
Let the Plan of Love and Light work out.
And may it seal the door where evil dwells.
Let Light and Love and Power restore the Plan on Earth. Amen

PRAYER PRIOR TO READING SCRIPTURE

Lord Jesus, open my eyes and my ears to Your Word.
That I may read and listen to Your voice,
and meditate on Your teachings.
Awaken my soul and my intelligence,
that Your Word penetrate my heart,
that I may savor it, and comprehend it.

Give me great faith in You,
that Your Words be for me lights that guide me through the paths of justice and truth.

Speak Lord, for I am listening, and desire to put to practice Your Doctrine, Because Your Word for me is joy, peace, and happiness. Speak Lord, Your are my Lord and my master, and I will not listen to anyone but You. Amen.

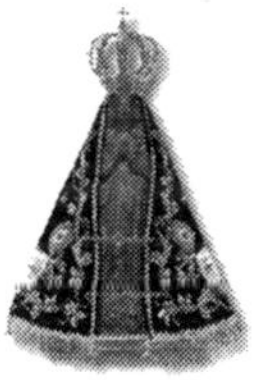

PRAYER TO OUR LADY NOSSA SRA. APARECIDA PATRONESS OF BRAZIL

Our Lady Aparecida, Patroness and Queen of Brazil, We thank You for your maternal protection.

Your children of Brazil implore Your protection against all types of violence and evil.

Help us obtain special graces, to help build a more just and fraternal nation, to live in true peace, and to someday find ourselves living in our definitive patrimony. Amen

PRAYER TO ARCHANGEL RAPHAEL FOR HEALTH

O Raphael of the glorious seven who stand before the throne of Him who lives and reigns. Angel of Health, the Lord hath filled thy hand with balm from Heaven to soothe or cure our pains. Heal or console the victims of disease; and guide our steps when doubtful of our ways. Amen

A PRAYER FOR A CLEAN HEART AND HEAVENLY WISDOM

Strengthen me O God, by the grace of Your Holy Spirit. Grant me the power to grow in holiness and to empty my heart of all useless care and anxiety. Give me Your heavenly wisdom, O Lord, that I may learn that the most important thing is to seek You and to find You, above all things to Love You. Amen.

PRAYER TO WORSHIP IN SPIRIT AND IN TRUTH

May we all learn to worship You in spirit, for You are spirit, and You have created us in Your image. May we all worship You by the Great Spirit of God that You are.

May we never have an idol in our lives—anyone or anything more important than You. May our worship be pleasing to You, and even in the midst of disappointment or great sorrow, may we always turn to You in worship.

Help us worship You in spirit and in truth—the truth of Who You are as You have revealed Yourself to be in the Scriptures—not the God we want You to be or imagine You are. Amen.

PRAYER OF THE ANGEL (THAT APPEARED AT FATIMA)

My God, I believe, I adore, I hope, and I love You. I implore Your pardon for those who do not believe, do not adore, do not hope, and do not love You. Most Holy Trinity - Father, Son, and the Holy Spirit - I adore You profoundly and offer You the most precious Body, Blood, Soul, and Divinity of Jesus Christ, present in all the tabernacles of the earth, in reparation for the outrages, sacrileges, and indifference by which He Himself is offended. And by the infinite merits of His most Sacred Heart and those of the Immaculate Heart of Mary, I beg of You the conversion of poor sinners.

Amen.

PRAYER TO THE SACRED FAMILY OF NAZARETH

Teach us to uplift each other,
teach us integrity and interiority.
Give us good disposition,
to listen to the great inspirations and
the words of the true masters.

Teach us the need of work,
of preparation, of the study of the interior life;
of prayer,
that only God sees in secret.

Teach us what is family,
its communion of love,
its beauty – simple and austere,

Its sacred and non-violent character. Amen.

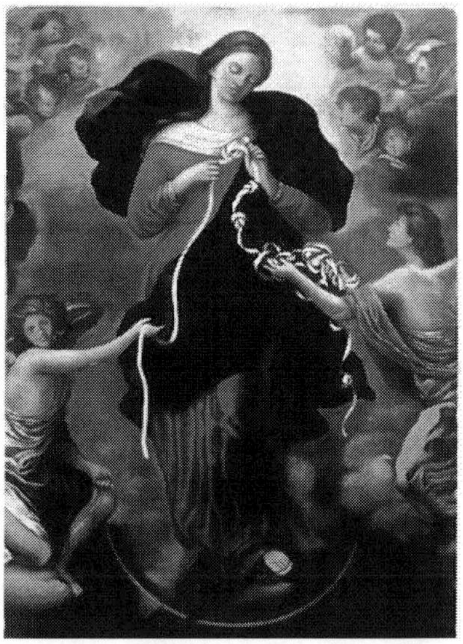

PRAYER TO OUR LADY DISSOLVER OF the KNOTS in OUR SOULS

Maria, undoer and dissolver of knots, untie the knot of depression (or culpability, anger, resentment, etc) in my soul.

Maria, undoer of knots, Maria of the God of life and Mother of those who are suffocated by anguish and are living in darkness, today I confide the knot of my depression (or culpability, anger, resentment....) to You.

Holy Mary, Mother of God, visit the house of my soul, poor and ill with this malady. You who brought the birthing sun to humanity, bring to me Your light so that I can again see the beauty of Life, and be uplifted with a new Spirit, that I may be able to smile, to sing, ...to love life and the Creator of my life.

Untie the knot of sadness and all that is dead inside of me because Your Son came to give me life – a life of abundance, to save all that is lost.

Just as you conceived Jesus, conceive with the Holy Spirit a new life for me.

Intercede for me close to Jesus, that the emptiness that I feel in my soul be filled with Your love and the love of whom loves me, without restrictions, and without end.

Consoling Angel, who consoled Jesus when His apostles abandoned Him, deliver this knot of my life to the Blessed Mother of God.

Maria, undoer and dissolver of knots, you whom made paradise reflourish, undo this knot so that I can reflourish for Jesus and find in Him the greatest reason to live and to be eternally grateful and happy. Amen

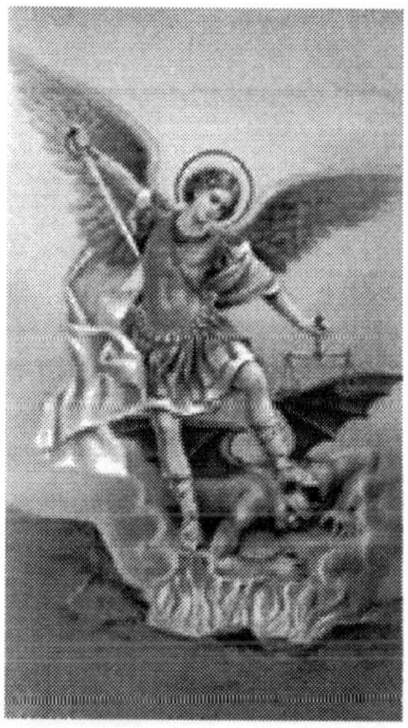

PRAYER TO ARCHANGEL MICHAEL FOR PROTECTION AND PERSEVERANCE

O God, Who made blessed Michael, thy Archangel, victorious over the proud Lucifer and all the wicked spirits, we beseech You that, fighting under the Cross and ever adopting his maxim, "Who is like unto God," we may be victorious over all our enemies and be delivered from all evils. Do regulate our lives according to Thy Will and Commandments, Through Jesus Christ our Lord. Amen

AN INTERFAITH PRAYER

O Creator Lord, let me feel the "isness" of things and people.

May He who is the Lord in Heaven of the Christians,
The Holy One of the Jews,
Allah of the Muslims,
Buddha of the Buddhists,
Tao of the Chinese,
Ahura Mazda of the Zoroastrians,
and Brahman of the Hindus
lead us from the unreal to the real,
from darkness to light,
from disease and death to immortality. Amen

LOVING KINDNESS MEDITATION

May all beings know happiness,
May all beings know love,
May all beings be wisely supported,
May all beings be free,
May all beings experience awakening!

A PRAYER FOR THOSE WHO SUFFER

For those who suffer and those who cry this day,
give relief from their burdens dear Lord.

Let them experience Your True peace.
Love them Lord, when others cannot.
Hold them Lord, when human arms fail.
Hear their prayers, O Lord,
and let them hear Your word of peace in their lives.
Amen

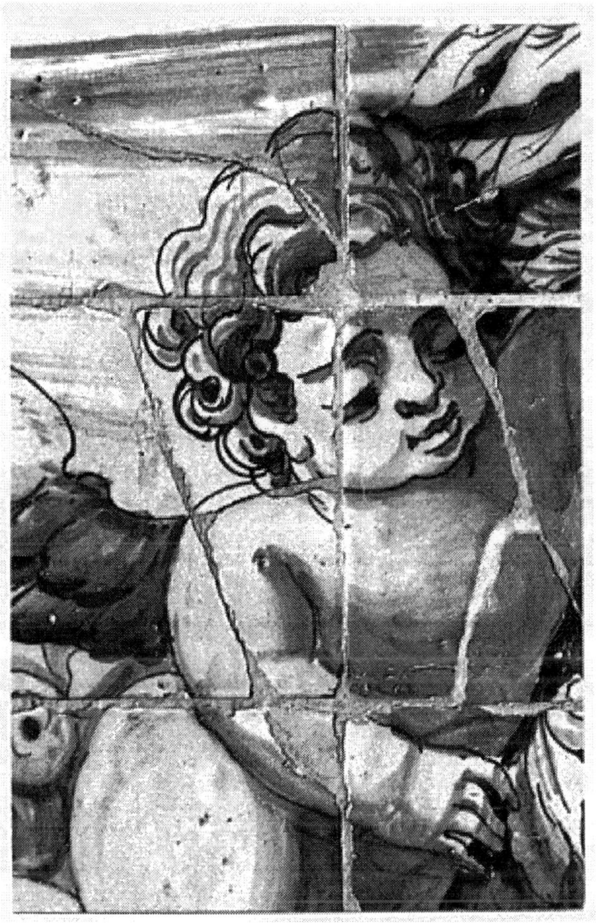

PRAYER TO THE NINE CHOIRS OF ANGELS

After each prayer recite a Glory Be (Glory Be to the Father, the Son, and the Holy Spirit as it was in the beginning, is now, and ever shall be, world without end, Amen.)

1) Oh, Holy creatures, pure Angels, noble spirits, ambassadors of the Glory and the Kingdom of God Almighty, and faithful executors of His orders, I beg of you to purify the prayer that I offer His Majesty, and bless it with light, faith, hope, and charity.

2) Oh, Faithful Archangels, captains of the celestial army, obtain for us, the light of the Holy Spirit and fortify us against the enemy.

3) Oh, sublime Authorities, governors of the world, govern us, that we may not be dominated by our senses.

4) Oh, Invincible Powers, restrain the malignant one when it assaults us and keep it from us, that it does not keep us from God.

5) Oh, Powerful Virtues, fortify our spirits, that full of your courage we can advance in the conquering of all virtues and resist all assaults of the evil one.

6) Oh, All Blessed Dominions, use your celestial forces to obtain for us perfect self-discipline, and perfect strength so that we can walk away from all that displeases God.

7) Oh, stable Throne of Eternity show unto all men the true path of eternal life, that we all prepare the dominion of the Lord that remains among all men.

8) Oh, Wise Cherubims, keep us in contemplation, that we always know the Greatness of the Lord.

9) Oh, Glowing Serafims, light us with your fire so that we love only those that you love incessantly.

ANCIENT HINDU PRAYER

We meditate on the transcendental Glory of the Deity Supreme, who is inside the heart of the earth, inside the life of the sky and inside the soul of the Heaven. May He stimulate and illuminate our minds. Lead us from the unreal to the real. Lead us from darkness to light. Lead us from death to immortality.

MAYAN PRAYER TO THE CREATOR

May thy heart be in the heart of the Universe.
May the heart of the universe be in my heart.
May my heart be in the heart of the Earth.
May the heart of Earth be in my heart.

PRAYER TO THE INFANT JESUS DURING DIFFICULT TIMES

I have a thousand difficulties: help me.

Of the enemies of my soul: save me.

In my poor judgments: illuminate me.

In my doubts and in my sorrows: comfort me.

In my solitude: accompany me.

In my illnesses: fortify me.

When they look down upon me: animate me.

In all temptations: defend me.

In my difficult hours: console me.

With Your Paternal heart: love me.

With Your immense power: protect me.

And in Your arms, as I expire: receive me. Amen

PRAYER TO DR. ADOLFO BEZERRA DE MENEZES FOR HIS INTERCESSION

Father of infinite justice and goodness, we beg of You with the help of Jesus and His legion of spiritual workers, in particular the benevolent and superior spirit of Dr. Adolfo Becerra de Menezes, that he assist us Lord, consoling the afflicted, curing those deserving your grace, comforting those experiencing difficult trials, discernment to those seeking Your truth, and assisting all those who appeal to Your infinite love and mercy.

Jesus, extend Your divine arms in aid of all who recognize You as their loyal and prudent dispensary. Make him (Becerra de Menezes), a divine model, through Your consoling legions, and superior spirits, in order that faith survive, hope increases, goodness expands, and love triumph over all things.

Becerra de Menezes, Apostle of peace and goodness, friend of the sick and humble, mobilize your assistants in benefit of those who suffer, whether they suffer from physical or spiritual maladies.

Good spirits, dignant workers of the Lord Almighty, shed heavenly cures throughout this suffering humanity, so that all creatures become friends with true knowledge and peace, forgiveness and harmony, sowing throughout the world the divine teachings of our Lord Jesus Christ. Amen.

PSALM 23 (for Provision)

The LORD is my shepherd, I shall not be in want. He makes me lie down in green pastures, He leads me beside quiet waters, He restores my soul. He guides me in paths of righteousness for His name's sake.

Even though I walk through the valley of the shadow of death, I will fear no evil, for You are with me; Your rod and Your staff, they comfort me.

You prepare a table before me in the presence of my enemies. You anoint my head with oil; my cup overflows. Surely goodness and love will follow me all the days of my life, and I will dwell in the house of the LORD forever. Amen.

PSALM 91 (for Protection)
ABIDING IN THE SHADOW OF THE ALMIGHTY

He who dwells in the shelter of the Most High

Will rest in the shadow of the Almighty.

I will say of the LORD,

He is my refuge and my fortress, my God in whom I trust.

Surely he will save you from the fowler's snare

and from the deadly pestilence.

He will cover you with his feathers,

and under his wings you will find refuge;

His faithfulness shall be your shield and rampart.

You will not fear the terror by night, nor the arrow that flies by day;

nor for the pestilence that stalks in the darkness,

nor for the plague that destroys at midday.

A thousand may fall at your side, ten thousand at your right hand; but it will not come near you.

You will only observe with your eyes

and see the punishment of the wicked.

If you make the Most High your dwelling – even the Lord who is my refuge

then no harm will befall you,

no disaster will come near your tent.

For he will command his angels

concerning you to watch you in all your ways:

they will lift you up in their hands, so that you will

not strike your foot against a stone.

You will tread upon the lion and the cobra;

you will trample the Great Lion and the serpent.

“Because he loves me,” says the Lord, “I will rescue him; I will protect him, for he acknowledges my name.”

He will call upon me, and I will answer him;

I will be with him in trouble,

I will deliver him and honor him.

With long life I will satisfy him and show him my salvation.

HEALING PRAYER AT BEDTIME

Lord Jesus, Through the Power of the Holy Spirit, go back into my memory as I sleep, every hurt that has ever been done to me, heal that hurt.

Every hurt that I have ever caused another person, heal that hurt. All the relationships that have been damaged in my whole life that I am not aware of, heal those relationships.

But Lord, if there is anything that I need to do, if I need to go to a person because he or she is still suffering from my hand, bring to my awareness that person, I choose to forgive and I ask to be forgiven. Remove whatever bitterness may be in my heart, Lord, and fill the empty spaces with Your Love. Amen

ST. FRANCIS OF ASSISI'S PRAYER

LORD, make me an instrument of Your peace.

Where there is hatred, let me sow love,

Where there is injury, pardon,

Where there is doubt, faith,

Where there is despair, hope,

Where there is darkness, light,

And where there is sadness, joy.

Divine Master, grant that I may not so much seek to be consoled as to console,

To be understood as to understand,

To be loved as to love,

For it is in giving that we receive,

It is in pardoning that we are pardoned, and it is in dying that we are born to eternal life. Amen

THE PRAYER OF THE GLASS OF WATER

The prayer begins with The Our Father, and continues "Holy Master, Physician of all physicians, turn your compassionate eyes to our ailing fellow men, whose names can be found in the LGW's Holy Book of Prayers: all those Brethren whom we think of in the hour of the Legionary Family's great vibration, Our Lord, You have said: " Ask, and GOD shall give to you. Not even towards the birds' death is GOD indifferent. Would any of you give your son a stone when he asks you for bread? Or would you give him a snake when he asks you for a fish? As bad as you are, you know to give good things to your children. How much more, then will your Father in Heaven, give good things to those who ask Him? This is why, Lord we want to ask You to place in this glass of water the perfect medicine for each one of us. That medicine you placed in the waters of the Jordan, or the waters of Siloe. That Celestial Medicine which recovered the sight of a blind-born man. We ask of you Our Holy Physician, place in this glass of water the Celestial Medicine for each one of us. May these ailing Brothers and Sisters whom we think of, sick in their bodies and sick in their souls, may they receive at this very moment the Blessing of Your cure, through the strength of this chain, in the name of GOD. Thank You, Lord! Give us the Divine Peace You have promised to those who live according to your New Commandment – My Peace I leave with you, My Peace I give unto you. Not as the world does, for I do not give you the Peace of the world. I give you the Peace of God, which the world cannot give. Let not your heart be troubled or afraid. For I will be with you, each and every day, until the end of the world! GLORY TO GOD IN THE HIGHEST AND PEACE ON EARTH TO ALL MEN AND WOMEN OF THE GOOD WILL OF GOD!"

PRAYER TO ST. EXPEDITUS FOR AN URGENCY

Noble Roman Youth, martyr, you who quickly brings things to pass, you who never delays, I come to you in need. -(state your need)-

Do this for me, St. Expeditus, and when it is accomplished, I will as rapidly reply for my part with an offering to you. – (state your promise)-

Be quick, St. Expeditus! Grant my wish before your candle burns out, and I will magnify your name. Amen

AN ANCIENT PRAYER OF DEVOTION

Jesus, may all that is you flow into me.
May Your body and blood unite me to yourself.
May Your passion and death be my strength and life.
Jesus, with you by my side enough has been given.
May the shelter I seek be the shadow of Your cross.
Let me not run from the love which You offer,
But hold me safe from the forces of evil.
On each of my dyings shed Your light and Your love.
Keep calling to me until that day comes when with Your saints, I may praise You forever. Amen.

BLESSING OF ST. JOSEPH

May the poverty of my sweet and suffering little Child be your riches; His sighs and tears, the consolation of your days; the love of His infant Heart, all your earthly treasure; and the clear vision of His adorable and glorified humanity, your eternal joy and recompense.

Amen.

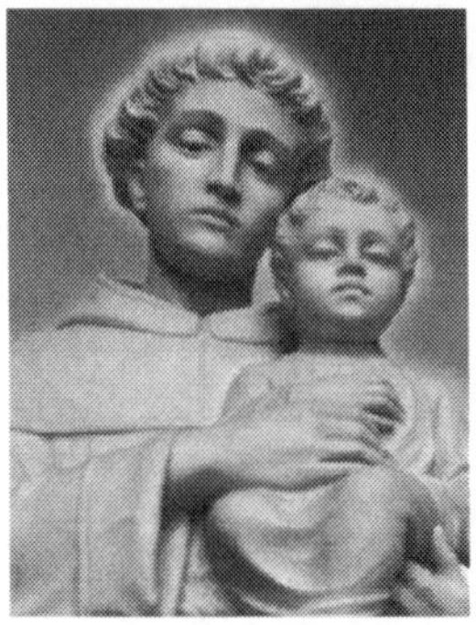

THE NINE GEMS OF THE CROWN OF ST ANTHONY

After each of the following prayers recite an Our Father, Hail Mary, and Glory Be.

1) The Sapphire of Faith – St. Anthony, Apostolic preacher and defender of the Christian faith, intercede for me, that I may conserve my faith as simple as a child, and with the courage and conviction which God has given me.

2) The Esmerald of Trust in God – Saint Anthony, great miracle worker because of your trust in God, reach for me a great distrust in myself and in my will and instead reach for me a limitless trust in God's power, will, and mercy.

3) The Ruby of the Love of God – St. Anthony, Seraphim of pure Divine love, reach for me the grace to always and above all things to love God, and to adhere to His commandments and to His will.

4) The Opal of Fraternal Love – St. Anthony, genuine imitator of the Great Samaritan, intercede for me, that I may comply with God's will, while loving others as well as myself.

5) The Topaz of Humanity – St. Anthony, mirror of humility and patience, grant me the grace of imitating thy example, overcoming pride and presumptuousness, and suffering with patience all the ills of this life.

6) The Amethyst of Mortification – St. Anthony, model of interior and exterior mortification, intercede for me, that I may overcome all passions and other inclinations, and produce fruits of a legitimate penitence.

7) The Diamond of the Strength of Perseverance – St. Anthony, courageous and victorious warrior of Jesus Christ, grant me the grace to always speak the truth and to conserve myself in it throughout eternity.

8) The Chrysolite of the Purity of Heart – St. Anthony, treasure of all virtues, intercede for me, grant that I may be granted freedom from all danger and all mortal sin.

9) The Pearl of Chastity – St. Anthony, angel of purity, grant me the grace from God that my body, mind, and soul remain free of sin, that I may one day deserve to see thy crown in heaven. Amen

PRAYER FOR THE TENDEREST HEART

My prayer is not for a share of the things the world calls great; but for the power to help some other on to a higher and happier state. Amen.

GLOSSARY

Affirmation is a form of therapeutic prayer. An affirmation helps crush limited and damaging thoughts and replaces them with positive and constructive ones.

Angelic Beings are celestial beings of light that inspire and protect humanity. They remind humans of their spiritual origin.

Aura is the body's exterior human energy system. It is the human envelope of light. The lighter and brighter the aura, the greater it reflects the individual's state of wholeness. The darker, denser aura reveals an individual that has lost touch with his soul and the cosmos, meaning there is an absence of love and light in his soul.

Balance/Equilibrium is the principle-healing objective in natural healing. It is centering oneself against the universe. It has to do with balancing the demands of this world with the reality of eternal life. When this is achieved we feel good about ourselves, we are happy, balanced, and at peace.

Buddhism is not a religion, but a way of life. Buddhist teachings include concepts of karma, reincarnation, self-responsibility, mindfulness, meditation and liberation, by way of detachment of material things.

Candomblé is the belief system that came from Africa, the Yoruba culture, and is strongly influenced by stories of *orixás* (spirits). In Rio de Janeiro it is known as Macumba and Umbanda, and in Recife as Xango.

Chakras are the interior human energy system They are seven interior wheels of light. It is a vortex of energy within the body. From the bottom up they are: The Root Chakra (grounding), Sacral Chakra (relationships), Solar Plexus Chakra (personal power), Heart Chakra ((love and compassion), Throat Chakra (communication), Third Eye Chakra (intuition), and the Crown Chakra (divine wisdom).

Charity is the science of human progress. It is helpfulness; a compromise with God and others to serve, particularly the poor, and those who suffer. It is a human obligation to the service of love, helping and comforting others. It is the greatest edifying therapy as it is love put into action, making constructive progress in the good of all humanity. It is a way of loving thy neighbor as thyself.

Clarity is our interior guiding light; leading us to what is naturally correct to do, clears away confusion. The brightness or dullness of our interior light depends on how much we think, feel, and act on the needs of the world.

Compassion is fervent brotherly love that stimulates a genuine concern. It is human moral responsibility. It is mindfulness that helps us live a virtuous human life. It empowers weak individuals without humiliating, criticizing, ridiculing, or harming them. Compassionate acts are generated and energized by love. Nature, the greatest compassion, very graciously allows the sinner plenty of time for repentance and retribution.

Consciousness is awareness and reverence for life. It is the level of intensity, of depth one wishes to live by. It is living life in constant relationship to the future, allowing each moment to have a balance against eternity rather than one short lifespan. Refers to human contact, human caring that drives us in the path of ripeness, productivity, brotherhood, love, peace, joy, and harmony. Consciousness is human concern and it cultivates moderation in life.

Contemplation is the profound examination that is required to reflect, plan, and put order (or reorder) in one's interior life.

Cosmology is the science of the universe. It is the study of the primary cosmic constituents, such as the origin and history of the chemical elements, and of space and time that form the frame of the expanding universe.

Cosmovision is a vision that requires an expansion (growth) of the spirit.

Courage requires a firm base of confidence, a deep-rooted trust and unshakeable faith that God is always present. Courage is needed to overcome obstacles in one's path and to effectively deal with personal struggles in life.

Desolation refers to an anguished soul. It is a soul in distress and sorrow. Part of human pain and suffering, this is the indication that a being is out of sync with nature and with cosmic harmony.

Detachment is the deprivation of the desire for all material things in exchange for the pursuit of all heavenly gifts. It helps us surrender to Divine will, to renounce self for God and for others.

Disincarnate is the soul without a body, or spirit being, an entity.

Discernment is avoiding deceit by synthesizing information and knowledge. It is the critical mindset needed for identifying truth from falsehood. The Spiritual Exercises (of St. Ignatius de Loyola) help individuals become more critical or discerned in identifying the nature of spirit entities; in identifying truth from falsehood. Becoming more discerned also helps individuals identify what God's purpose is for them.

Disobsession Procedures is a type of moral psychiatric medicine that heals the unbalanced state of the mind caused by spirit obsessors. This is done during a mediumship meeting where counselors converse with the manifesting entities in their attempt to enlighten the unhappy disincarnate spirit(s) that continue to live in mental darkness. The healing occurs when both the obsessor and the patient are released from each other after the obsessor spirit is counseled to let go of the incarnate soul and is instructed to follow the Light. Common obsessive conditions are depression, anorexia, obesity, phobias, any compulsive and obsessive behavior, such as sexual addiction and obsession, drug addictions, kleptomania, rape, and criminal behavior.

Disorder in life causes illness. The order or disorder of the exterior life reflects the order or disorder of the inner life.

Distant/Remote Healing is healing that is done from a distance. Here distance is not space it is only a degree of perception.

Ecumenical refers to religious tolerance, finding unity, universality in religious experience. Requires a communal mindset. Seeking the spirit of God in everything and everyone.

Electromagnetic Fields refers to the fields throughout the electromagnetic spectrum. A changing electric field always produces a magnetic field. The interaction between both of these forces (electric and magnetic) creates a new condition in space, the electromagnetic field.

Emotions are a form of energy. Negative emotions play an important role in the creation of blocked energies, thus creating an accumulation of wasted energy in a corresponding organ or chakra. Positive emotions help maintain balanced energy – help sustain optimal health.

Emotional illness is illness that is caused by becoming despondent to the needs of others, to the social injustices, inequities, and oppression that prevail.

Energy refers to the strength of God, God's vitality in humankind.

Energy Vibrations see intuition.

Enlightenment is a spiritual reawakening. It is a new-found faculty of inner sight, a new profoundness or depth of our existence, as we know it. To be born into light requires finding one's courage.

Entity is a spirit being, a disincarnate soul.

Esoteric is the "inner" (eso-), in the sense of the inner consciousness, the contemplative, mystical, and meditative transpersonal perspective. Only intuition, or higher mental or spiritual faculties can help understand the esoteric experience.

Eternal knowledge is the essence of all things and all beings. It helps avoid crystallizing human thoughts, ideas, bad habits, and harmful conditioning.

Etiology is the science that deals with the causes or origins of disease.

Evolution emerges from the Law of Ripeness, spiritual evolution is about our spiritual consciousness expanding, growing, maturing, fully ripening thus bringing one forth from a lesser to a greater self. It is positive change.

Expiation and Reparation of sins help recreate a new expression of oneself. Forgiving is a start, but expiation and reparation are necessary to recreate a new beginning, a new energy.

Faith is our greatest power. It is one's confidence, firmness, or integrity of being in sacred unity. It has been spoiled as it has been put on a unique platform. It is complete trust in God. Trust in God goes wherever life takes you, particularly the unknown. It is the opposite of fear.

Fasting is a deeply felt sacrifice, more than the absence of food in the stomach. It is generally a reduction of food consumption, done in the spirit of atonement.

Fear is the opposite of faith. It is a most crippling element**.** It is fright, apprehension, and anxiety. Fear is also extreme reverence toward a superior power.

Fluidized Magnetized Water is water that has been blessed or meditated upon, and has received heaven's medicinal balm through the radiations of a healer's best energies. The vibrations during the 22nd hour (10pm) are the most appropriate to solicit the most powerful and purified fluidized water from the spiritual plane.

Forgiveness is the release of an injury done against us or done by us. By forgiving the restoration process begins. It is essential to revert to the original state of wholeness in order that positive change take place.

Gnosticism is a way of understanding, higher than reason alone. Gnostics speak of their God as Father-Mother-Son (all in one). The path of the Gnostics in the early centuries of Christianity, was salvation through self-knowledge, enlightenment in union with God. They taught their members a path to "the place of peace within."

Gospel is the teachings or the doctrine of a religious leader. It refers to the proclamation of the redemption preached by Jesus and His Apostles. Clear and simple, it is the teachings of unity of God and Man to humanity.

Health is a multidimensional phenomenon that involves physical, psychological, social and spiritual aspects. It is the harmony and balance of the individual.

Healing refers to the attunement of healing energies that are granted to patients with imbalances or deficiencies in order that their vital centers be reactivated, their equilibrium restored, and their complete health recovered.

Healing Mediums provide treatments that respond to the patient's wider social, cultural, and cosmic realities with the help of the spirit world. They encourage their patients to embark on a path of self-discovery by individual efforts of work, study, and good works.

Heresy is any opinion or doctrine that contradicts any Orthodox doctrines or teachings.

Higher Self can be thought of as the soul, the point of contact with the Creator and the spirit world. By nature it is free of mundane limitations.

Hinduism is regarded as the oldest of the organized religions. It is now the third largest religion in the world, even after breaking off into thousands of religions in more than 3500 years. A central pillar is the belief of karma and reincarnation.

Holy, inwardly refers to all that is pure, and outwardly, all that is noble. It is the profound engagement between all life forms. It is respect for the spirit in everything. The aim of a Holy person is to serve, praise, and venerate God and all of His creation, in humility and away from self-centered attachments. It is seeing the sacredness and divinity in all.

Holy Eucharist is a Christian sacrament, which was instituted by Christ during His last supper with the apostles. It is a ritual of communion with God and Christ, where bread and wine are consecrated and consumed in remembrance of Christ.

Holy Rosary is a form of voluntary prayer used primarily by Catholics and Christians. The way it is prayed today began with Saint Dominic who received a vision and a rosary from the Blessed Mother of God instructing him to pray in order to save souls and convert sinners. It is composed of the mysteries of the lives of Jesus and Mary. The term “rosary” derived from the Mystical Rose term given to the Blessed Virgin Mary.

Homeopathic Medicine is a medical approach that respects the wisdom of the body. It utilizes medicines that stimulate the body’s own immune and defense systems in healing.

Human Energy Field is the manifestation of the cosmic energy that is intimately involved with human life. It is the energy field that surrounds the human body, also known as the human aura, the vital force in humans.

Illness is a disintegration of the organic, psychological, and spiritual bodies. Ailments of the soul can only be treated with spiritual therapy. From the spiritual viewpoint illness could be the product of a repressed character, a neglected past that requires attention, reorganization, and balance.

Imagination is a very powerful transmuting chemical. It promises to take one beyond the limits of one’s present conceptions, and present experiences. It has the power to heal open wounds that no therapy has the ability to heal.

Immortality of the Soul refers to eternal life. The soul never dies, only the physical body.

Incarnate refers to the soul living within the physical body. To be physically alive.

Indulgence refers to the remission of temporal punishment still due for a sin that has been absolved. Prayer and works of charity are considered indulgences.

Inertia is atrophied force; a loss of productivity. It is shutting oneself from the current that gives life force and intensity. It is the same as being indifferent, inactive, or despondent.

Inner Peace refers to the peace of God within us, it helps us feel genuinely human.

Intention is the foresight of a particular consequence before it manifests.

Integrative Medicine is medicine that integrates, unifies, brings together, and makes whole again. It is medicine that cooperates, collaborates with other medical systems, healing and spiritual traditions.

Intercessory Prayer is an intention filled with love and goodness and is manifested with radiations of our best energies. Assists others and has a healing effect.

Intuition is a vibratory field involving perception beyond the senses. It is the voice from the spirit realm, the voice that leads to the discovery of new things. One must be open to receive perception that is divinely inspired. Intuition becomes blocked with toxins, negative emotions, and inertia.

Jesuit is an order of the Catholic Church, also known as the Society of Jesus, founded by St. Ignatius de Loyola. It's principle goal is to spread God's love through the world, by way of education and service.

Judeo-Christian is of historical relationship to Judaism and early Christian traditions.

Kardecist teachings have helped establish important principles of communication between the physical and spiritual worlds. Are bridging the gap between religion, philosophy, and science.

Karma is cosmic obligation to oneself and to the universe. It is about encouraging a review of one's belief system and putting it in harmony with the universe, so that one may be *released* from past karma. It is the scale that balances our energy, takes care of any imbalances. In Physics it is known as the Law of Compensation, The Law of Balance, or the Law of Justice. It is receiving what one has earned, reaping what one has sown by means of encouragement.

Law of Cause and Effect in biblical terms refers to "As you sow, so you shall reap." It is the universal equalizer. For every action there will be an equal reaction. AKA, Law of Attraction.

Law Of Selfless and Unconditional love supercedes all Laws. Love empowers. It is the oxygen of the soul – it is the energy of life. The more it is divided, and more it is given away, the stronger and greater it becomes.

Law Of Ripeness cultivates the seed of life that takes one from the lesser self to the greater self. The seed must mature to the next stage, if not, it will rot. It is the same as the natural Law of Evolution.

Law of Right is the highest of God's laws; mercy stands above all statute laws.

Life is eternal and cyclical. It takes place with or without a body. With a body we call it "alive," without it we call it "death." Spiritists contend there is one eternal life, with numerous physical incarnations and spiritual disincarnations.

Love is the creating and maintaining substance of the universe. Just as air is indispensable for organic existence, love is indispensable as it is the oxygen of the soul.

Magnetic (Physical) Passes are emanations conducted by physical beings that aid patients in restoring physical health via the exchange of magnetic fluids between patient and healer. This exchange does not involve a spirit entity. The first steps in establishing this method of healing in the 18th century, is credited to a German physician Franz Anton Mesmer.

Mandala is an aid to meditation. It is a geometric design of the universe, a ritualistic tool used in early eastern religions.

Mantra is a transcendental sound or a vedic hymn. It is used in an effort to empty the mind in meditation and to obtain consciousness. Promotes healing.

Medical Anthropology is the academic field that looks at the way individuals have approached issues of health, illness, and healing in their respective ways, across all cultures, and throughout time.

Medical Spiritist Association is a professional Brazilian organization aiming to construct a new generation of integrative health professionals to create the world's first transcendental and humanistic model of medicine.

Meditation is the conscious contact with the source of life. It is the loss of contact with our human sensory currents that go beyond the ego, in order to find moderation, harmony, and balance in life. Meditation does not prevent difficult things from occurring; instead it helps individuals deal with them.

Mediums are masters of spirits that can help those who have gone astray find their way onto their spiritual path.

Mediumship is a psychobiological predisposition inherent to those who under certain conditions are allowed to capture the thoughts of disincarnate spirits, experience the astral plane, and establish contact with the spirit world.

Mental illness is an impairment of a person's cognitive, emotional, or behavioral functioning. Spiritual healers believe the cause could be a spirit attachment, obsession, and could also be of social, genetic, psychological, or biochemical origin.

Meridians are a part of a network of channels in the human body that are responsible for the circulation of vital energy.

Mind-Body-Spirit is about a trilogy – three major components of the human experience. It is about regenerating the energy fields of all three to obtain optimal health, holistic health.

Mindfulness is true concern. It is control of self. A gentle reminder from God for one to think, feel, and do for others before thinking, feeling and doing for oneself.

Miracle is a supernatural event, meaning it is only accomplished with divine intervention.

Moral Flab refers to an unkept, undisciplined soul. It is spiritual laziness that cripples self-expression, hinders the ability to look beyond oneself, represses the human spiritual nature of mankind, and robs one of a complete human experience. Moral flab creates confusion, inertia, and spiritual ignorance.

Morality equips one with mindfulness and consciousness. Guarding one's mindfulness is essential in living an ethical life. It is a code of ethics that helps one find happiness and avoid suffering.

Multifaith refers to a new community of people from all faiths coming together to celebrate the many faces of God, celebrating true unity in God.

Mysteries of Faith in Catholicism and Christianity refers to the mystical life events of Jesus Christ and His mother, the Blessed Virgin Mary. They are the Joyous, Sorrowful, Glorious, and Luminous Mysteries that teach us about the Life, Passion, Crucifixion, Death, and Resurrection of Christ and His Blessed Mother who was with Him during each of these important life and death events.

Mystic is someone who believes life to be more than physical or material. A mystic believes in a reality that is of the spirit realm.

Mysticism is any philosophy whose roots are in mystical experience, intuitions, or direct experiences of the Divine. In such experiences the mystic believes that his or her soul has temporarily achieved union with God.

Obsession is a condition that requires spiritual treatment, behavior change, and inner transformation. In severe cases it may cause physical and mental ailments (see disobsession procedures).

Obsessor in spiritism is referred to a spiritual entity that attaches itself to a person for the purpose of causing anxiety, confusion, depression, and suffering. Most often the obsessor is someone known to the patient from a previous relationship gone wrong (from this incarnation or a prior one). The principle objective of an obsessor is to hinder the patient's evolutionary growth.

Oracle is a person who can see into the future, one who can prophecy. An infallible truth given by a priest or priestess; it also refers to a temple where a prophet is in communication with God.

Order is eternal and maintains harmony. When things are out of order, the natural balance of life, losses synchrony, becoming unhappy or ill. This happens because the natural order of things in the universe has been altered.

Orthodox/Conventional refers to an unquestionable doctrine or religious teaching. A teaching that is traditionally and blindly accepted.

Paradigm is a classification. A fitting into a certain pattern or model.

Parapsychology involves the study of extrasensory perception in psychological phenomenon such as clairvoyance, telepathy, psycho-kinesis, etc.

Passionflower is an herbal supplement that is used to tranquilize anxiety and nervousness. It helps promote sleep. Its spirit energy evokes divine consciousness.

Perispirit is the subtle body around the human body made up of the universal cosmic fluid. The spirit to connect to the perceptions of the human brain uses the perispirit.

Personal Transformation involves an improvement of the soul, mind, and physical being.

Power to Create enables one to transcend through time and space – always in constant relationship to the future. It is the point where one can connect beyond one's experiences, beyond one's present human limitations and inferior way of thinking.

Prayer is talking with God. It is a profound expression of gratitude for all of one's experiences (joys, abundance, and losses). With prayer one learns to cultivate gratitude, discipline, moderation, humility, detachment, readiness, preparedness, and spiritual protection. It is the tool that best helps one form an interior and exterior life, taking one from the lesser to the greater self.

Psychic is a person who is sensitive to the energies emanating from another individual's aura. Using these energies mostly with clairvoyance, intuition, and divination.

Psychotherapy is the treatment of emotional and mental disorders. In biomedicine psychological techniques are applied to open communication between therapist and patient that can lead the patient to better functioning.

Purification of the soul is done by forgiving and performing good works of charity. Both cleanse consciousness and clarify how one perceives the world. Purifying negative karma should be done before it manifests as suffering. Only a pure soul can be the foundation of spiritual mastership. The vessel must be cleansed before pouring the water of life into it.

Quantum Physics is the branch of physics that uses the quantum theory (using discrete indivisible units of energy) to explain the properties of a physical system.

Radiations are a form of telepathic transmissions. They are mental and fluidic emanations, such as mental emanations of strength, courage, and trust that are projected and received by another individual.

Reason is the human capacity for rational, logical, analytical thinking. Reason does not know how to deal with pain or how to explain it, as it requires a transcendental and mystical explanation.

Reincarnation refers to the soul's progression through eternity until it reaches the fullness of eternal life in God. It is the rebirth of the soul, the wheel of birth, death and rebirth. For the incarnate and disincarnate soul, its final goal is to be liberated from karma after reaching triumphantly, entry into God's Kingdom (the home of the soul).

Religion is a strong cultural element that practices ritual and worship of the Creator. Organized religion and even those religions that claim not to be organized, pass on to their members, divine and codified teachings. These aim to provide direction, order, and structure. Religion motivates all aspects of human behavior, as it is an important cultural element.

Resurrection as interpreted by biblical scholars is coming back to life from physical death, being reborn to a new physical life.

Reverence is love, respect, honor, and devotion to God, everyone and everything around us. It is also tolerance for other's individual differences.

Ritual is a meeting that symbolizes and reproduces creation. It is a non-verbal way of enacting the purpose and meaning of life and death. Rituals provide depth to human understanding. In religious context, ritual is a diligent call to worship particularly to commemorate a significant life-of-passage event (e.g. birth, puberty, marriage, and death). Rituals normally are commemorated among members of the community elevating the rank of importance to a greater one.

Sacred is the highest degree of respect for God, all beings, and all things. Sacredness helps cultivate gratitude and moderation.

Saints are humans who have led extraordinary and exemplary lives of sacrifice, piety, humility, service, devotion, and temperance. Humans can call upon their spirit for intercession with a special prayer request to be presented before the Creator.

Salvation in scriptures refers to giving life-energy to someone, to empower them by saving their soul.

Self-Realization is the fulfillment of one's potential. In Hinduism it refers to the culmination of all things spiritual, the final release of the cycle of life and rebirth.

Self-Responsibility is the awareness every person has about their responsibility in the consequences of their own decisions and their own health.

Sinner is one who has gone against God's will, has broken the Laws of God. It is someone who is spiritually dead, who has fallen into error; who lives in the shadow of ignorance and who needs restoration.

Social Irresponsibility has to do with a lack of enthusiasm for justice, making one numb to the many social injustices, inequities, and oppression that are alive today. Conformity has to do with becoming despondent to the needs of others. It is the opposite of being mindful.

Soul is the higher spiritual self. It is the vision from the point of origin, way beyond our present recollection. The soul carries the mental and spiritual capital and leaves the physical temporary capital behind. It is the extent of one's inner reality. The soul organizes, regenerates, and creates everything in its existence. It is the center of energy and carries man's ideals. The soul is the essence of eternal life.

Spirit is an intelligent being. Spirits are souls that no longer reside in the human body. Rather, they live in the spirit world after physical death. The soul and the spirit are the same entity - we call it soul when it is in the human body and we perceive it as being alive; we call it spirit when it is outside the body and we perceive it dead.

Spiritism is a way of life that provides a profound understanding of the human soul, humanity's purpose, and spiritual evolution, helping establish important scientific principles between the spiritual and physical worlds. As a science, Spiritism can be seen as the search of the truth of humanity's spiritual nature with the principle objective of helping humanity heal, progress, and evolve. It has opened new horizons for the study of many psychic phenomenon and has helped establish a scientific classification for mediumship (see Kardecist Teachings).

Spiritist (aka Kardecist), is someone who adheres to the philosophy that deals with the origin, nature, and destiny of spirits as well as their relationship with the corporeal world. Spiritists believe their practice is not one that communicates with the dead. Rather, they believe mediums communicate with the Spirit of Truth –

communicating concepts of truth that can offer lasting freedom to humanity.

Spiritual is of or pertaining to spirit, to the non-material. It refers to a natural yearning for God, an individual pursuit of truth, following the way. Spirituality encourages the seeker to venture out on the lonely and difficult path of self-knowledge. It is one's knowledge of God after extending one's knowledge of the world, and of oneself. It culminates in mindfulness, and a communal mindset.

Spiritual Consolation is love for God, a positive movement in the soul, the light and warmth of God in the soul. It involves surrendering one's will to God's will, allowing His will to penetrate one's thoughts, words, and deeds.

Spiritual Desolation is the darkness of a soul, has to do with lesser evolved, and lowly spirits influencing one's thoughts, words, and deeds.

Spiritual Education is illumination for the soul. It helps to avoid crystallizing human thoughts, ideas, habitual patterns, and harmful conditioning. It refers to exploring in degrees what we yet do not know and that which we wish to understand. To understand information more clearly it must not be dichotomized, instead it must be contextualized, viewing it as wisdom that is ripe. The aim of a spiritual education, is personal transformation, it is not to get caught up in the debates, nor to empower only oneself.

Spiritual Evolution is about the spirit growing, maturing, perfecting. It is a process of purification, and correction in getting closer to the perfection God is.

Spiritual Healing comes about from the direct contact between man and God.

Spiritual Health is the greatest of Divine treasures. It requires we maintain it with constant zeal, meditation, worship, justice, truth, and good works.

Spiritual Passes are emanations conducted by superior spirit beings through a healing medium and affect the organization of the patient's perispirit. Spiritual passes, coming from superior spirit beings, have greater healing power than magnetic passes (which are not done by spirit entities but rather physical beings).

Spiritual Reflection is about examining our discontents, not resenting them or enduring them, but examining them to resolve them. Reflection is the clarity of the eye of the soul, it helps clear out unnecessary baggage and helps put reorder back in its place.

Spiritual Traditions are spiritual practices that have been passed down through generations (such as ancestor worship, prayer, meditation, etc.). Their aim is to bring balance, peace, and harmony into one's life, by keeping one connected to the spirit world.

Spiritualist is someone who believes in a spiritual dimension beyond this visible and physical world. He may believe in the existence of spiritual beings, and may ask for their intercession, guidance and protection. In the American and British usage, spiritualist, is more clearly defined as a belief that the dead communicate with the living through mediums. Unlike spiritists, spiritualists may not believe in the concept of reincarnation.

Suffering refers to an anguished soul. It is a purification filter for clearing past negative karma. It also exists to serve as an active role in which it can help others better their souls.

Supernatural refers to anything that is not considered of the natural world. It involves the spirit world. It is not of the senses, but instead is of ultra-sensory perception.

Trabalhar is the Portuguese word for "work." In the spiritual sense it refers to the work done for the common good. It is the firm belief that one must be actively engaged in the construction of the kingdom of heaven on earth, before expecting to receive God's grace and mercy.

Trance is a semiconscious and detached state of being. A state of experiencing both worlds: physical and spiritual simultaneously.

Transcendental refers to a new superior model that surpasses all previous models.

Transpersonal psychology is the extension of psychological studies into consciousness studies, spiritual inquiry, body-mind relationships, and transformation.

Triangle in Christianity and Catholicism is a symbolic representation of God Triune (God the Father, God the Son, and God the Holy Spirit [the female aspect]). It is also representative of the fraternal brotherhood found in ancient eastern philosophies. Together with the fraternity of the cross (found in western thought which divulges the teachings of Christ), they symbolize the *unity* of God.

Truth liberates. It opens possibilities, and creates transformation through the renovation of the spirit. Truth is strong and vigorous as it keeps universal harmony. Truth is flawless as it is unchanging. However man's free will and intellectual powers can change people's perception of truth.

The Way refers to one's individual life path, one's individual bliss; a path that leads one to the truth and perfection with God.

Universal Life Force is a vital force or energy that transcends time and space. All beings and all things depend on it for their health and their life.

Unity is when two or more become one in thought, one in heart, one in family, and one in God. It is the Oneness in God and His creation.

Visualizations are therapeutic tools used in healing that use suggestive mental imagery.

Wellness refers to a happy disposition. With plenty of work, rest, a balanced diet, physical exercise, and spiritual education, wellness can be achieved.

Worship is human adoration of the Almighty Divine Spirit. It is time set aside to devoutly praise and honor the Creator; to give thanks for everything in one's life. Worship differs from veneration, which implies respect or honor for a spirit entity, such as a saint or angel that is called in fellowship to assist one with a prayer petition.

NOTES

NOTES

NOTES

NOTES

NOTES

READINGS FOR FURTHER STUDY

Armond, E. (1990). Passes e Radiaçoes: Metodos Espírita de Cura. Passes and Radiations: Spiritist Healing Methods. São Paulo: Editora Alianca.

Associação Médico-Espírita do Brasil. (2004). Saude e Espiritismo. Campos de força, mediunidade, sexualidade e abordagens na prática médica. Health and Spiritism: Fields of force, mediumship, sexuality, and approaches to medical practice. São Paulo: AME-Brasil.

Associação Médico-Espírita de Minas Gerais. (2004). Porque Adoeçemos (Novos horizontes do conhecimento médico-espírita). Why We Become Ill: New horizons in the the medical-spiritist understandings. São Paulo: AME-Brasil.

Associação Médico-Espírita de Minas Gerais. (2004). Porque Adoeçemos II. Principios para a medicina da alma. Why we Become Ill. Principles of medicine for the soul. São Paulo: AME-Brasil.

Bodine, E. (1985). Hands that Heal. Novato: New World Library.

Bragdon, E. PhD. (2002). Spiritual Alliances: Discovering the roots of health at the Casa de Dom Inácio. Woodstock: Lightening Up Press.

Bragdon, E. PhD. (2004). Kardec's Spiritism: A home for healing and spiritual evolution. Woodstock: Lightening Up Press.

Brennan, B.A. (1987). Hands of Light: A Guide to healing through the human energy field. New York: Bantam Books.

Brolio, Dr. R. (1999). Educaçao da Alma. Educating the Soul. São Paulo: FE Editora Jornalistica, Ltda.

Brolio, Dr. R. B. (2000). Doenças da Alma. Soul Illness. São Paulo: FE Editora Jornalistica, Ltda.

Co, S., & E.B. Robins. (2002). Your Hands can Heal You: pranic healing energy remedies to boost vitality and speed recovery from common health problems. New York: Free Press.

Costa de Araujo Lima, M. (1994). Parapsicologia: Da magia á ciência. Parapsychology: From magic to science. Porto Alegre: Editora Mercado Aberto Ltda.

Costa, V. R. (2001). Enfermedades Da Alma: e a proposta terapeutica espírita. Soul Illness: The proposed Spiritist therapy. Sao Paulo: DPL-Editora e Distribuidora de Livros, Ltda.

Douglas-Klotz, N. (1999). The Hidden Gospel: Decoding the Spiritual Message of the Aramaic Jesus. Wheaton: Quest Books.

Dossey, L. (1993). Healing Words. New York: Harper Paperbacks.

Emoto, M. (2001). The Hidden Messages in Water. Tokyo: Sunmark.

Estrich-Pellegrino, R. (2003). The Power to Heal: A concise and comprehensive guide to energy healing. Goiánia: Gráfica Terra.

Fabri dos Anjos, M. (2004). Novas Gerações e Vida Religiosa: Pesquisa e analyses prospectivas sobre a vida religiosa no Brasil. New Generations and Religious Life: Analysis and Research Perspectives on Religious Life in Brazil. Parecida: Editora Santuário.

Franco. D.P. (1998). Amor, Imbatível Amor. Love, Invincible Love. Salvador: Centro Espírita de Redenção.

Franco. D.P. (1991). Plenitude. Plenitude. Salvador: Centro Espírita de Redenção.

Gerber, R. (1996). Vibrational Medicine: New choices for healing ourselves. Santa Fe: Bear & Company.

Goswami, A. (2001). Physics of the Soul. Charlottesville: Hampton Roads.

Govinda, K. (2002). A Handbook of Chakra Healing: Spiritual practice for health, harmony, and inner peace. Old Saybrook: Konecky and Konecky.

Kulcheski, E. (2001). Os mecanismos da cura espiritual The mechanisms of a spiritual cure. Revista Crista de Espiritismo, 2, 8-11.

Larson, D., Milano, B., & Lu, F. (1988). Religion and mental health: The need for cultural sensitivity and synthesis. In: S. O. Okpaku (Ed.), Clinical methods in transcultural psychiatry (pp.191-210). Washington D.C.: American Psychiatric Press.

Leonesy Pontes, J. A. (1994). Esoterismo á Luz do Espiritismo. Esoterism the Light of Spiritism. Salvador: Gráfica Contraste.

Loyola, I. (2000). The Spiritual Exercises of St. Ignatius. New York: Random House.

Martin, B. (2000). Change Your Aura, Change Your Life: A step-by-step guide to unfolding your spiritual power. Sunland: Wisdom Light Books.

Matthews, D., M.D. & C. Clark (1998). The Faith Factor: Is Religion Good for Your Health? New York: Penguin Group.

Mishlove, J. (1993). Roots of Consciousness: Theory: The biological perspective. [Online]. Available at: http://www.williamjames.com/Theory/BIOLOGY.htm

Myss, C. PhD. (1996). Anatomy of the Spirit: The seven stages of power and healing. New York: Crown Publishers.

Netto, J.P. (1989). Spiritualistic Guidelines of the World LGW. Sao Paulo: Legion of Good Will.

Petersen, K. Laying On Of Hands. The Silva Method. [Online] Available at: http://www.silvamethod.com/rp/docs/hands.pdf

Schubert, S.C. (2004). Os Poderes da Mente. The Powers of the Mind. Sao Paulo: EBM Editora.

Sullivan, R. Hospitals Introducing a Therapy Resembling 'Laying On Of Hands'. The Silva Method. [Online] Available at: http://www.silvamethod.com/rp/docs/hands.pdf

Xavier, F.C. (1938). Brasil, Coraçao do Mundo Patria do Evangelho. Brazil, Heart of the World, Land of the Gospel. Rio de Janeiro: Federaçao Espirita Brasileira.

Xavier, F.C. (1944). The Astral City. Rio de Janeiro: Federaçao Espírita Brasileira.

Xavier, F.C. (1945). Missionários da Luz. Light Missionaries. Brasilia: Federaçao Espírita Brasileira.

Xavier, F.C. (1945). Os Mensageiros. The Messengers. Brasilia: Federaçao Espírita Brasileira.

Xavier, F.C. (1948). Christian Agenda. London: Clifford Frost Limited.

BIBLIOGRAPHY

Benson, H. (2000). The Relaxation Response. New York: Harpertorch.

Dowling, L. (1979). The Aquarian Gospel of Jesus the Christ. Marina del Rey: DeVorss & Co.

Epstein, D. (2007). Countries of the CARMEN Network for chronic disease prevention and control meet in Bahamas: PAHO Urges Pan American action to stop regional epidemic of chronic diseases. [Online]. Available at: http://www.paho.org/English/DD/PIN/pr071106a.htm

Estrich-Pellegrino, R. (1997). The Miracle Man: The life and story of João de Deus. Cairns, Queensland, Australia: Triad. Website: http://www.robertpellegrinoestrich.com

Finkler, K. (1994). Sacred healing and biomedicine compared. Medical Anthropology Quarterly 8(2), 178-197.

Goulding, M. (2007). Surgery and Pills Couldn't Help Me: A Brazilian shaman said he could. An adventure on the edge between medicine and miracles. [Online]. Available at: http://www.menshealth.com/cda/article.do?site=MensHealth&channel=health&category=doctors.hospit

als&conitem=25b7808f3eb34110VgnVCM1000001 3281eac____&page=1

Harvey, C., & Cochrane, A. (1999). The Healing Spirit of Plants: An illustrated guide to plant spirit medicine. New York: Sterling.

"Is John of God Healer or a Charlatan?: Searching for hope and health in a remote Brazilian village." ABC News. Host John Quiñones. February 10 2005.

[Online]. Available at: http://abcnews.go.com/Health/Primetime/story?id=482292&page=1

Kardec, A. (2003) The Spirit's Book. Philadelphia: Allan Kardec Educational Society.

Kardec, A. (2000). The Gospel Explained by the Spiritist Doctrine. Philadelphia: The Allan Kardec Educational Society.

Koenig, H., McCullough, M. & D. Larson (2001). Handbook of Religion and Health. New York: Oxford.

Krippner, S. (1987). Cross-cultural approaches to multiple personality disorder: Practices in Brazilian spiritism. Ethos, 15, 273-295.

Lerner, M. (2000). Spirit Matters. Charlottesville: Hampton Roads Publishing.

Mishlove, J. (1998). Psychic and spiritual healing with Stanley Krippner, Ph.D. [Online]. Transcript of an interview. Available at: http://www.intuition.org/txt/krippner.htm

RavenWing, J. (2002.) The Book of Miracles: The healing work of João de Deus. Fairfield: 1st Books. Website: http://www.healingjourneys.net

SEER (2007). (Surveillance Epidimiology and End Results) Annual Report to the Nation on the Status of Cancer, 1975–2004. [Online]. Available at: http://seer.cancer.gov/report_to_nation/

Smith, J. (1973). The influence of enzyme growth by the "laying on of hands." In California Academy of Parapsychology and Medicine (Ed.), Dimensions of healing: A symposium. Los Altos, Ca: California Academy of Parapsychology and Medicine

Starfield, B. (2000). Is the US Health really the best in the world? JAMA, 284 (4), 483-485.

Voeks, R. (1997). Sacred Leaves of Candomble: African magic, medicine, and religion in Brazil. Austin: University of Texas Press.

WHO Global InfoBase (2002). Deaths Caused by Malignant Neoplasms 2002 Brazil and US compared. [Online] Available at: http://www.who.int/infobase/compare.aspx?dm=10&countries=76%2c840&year=2002&sf1=mo.cg.059&sex=all

WHO Global InfoBase (2002). Mortality Deaths, Neuropsychiatric Conditions. [Online]. Available at: http://www.who.int/infobase/compare.aspx?dm=10&countries=76%2c840&year=2002&sf1=mo.cg.059&sex=3

WHOSIS, Brazil. (2002). Brazil Mortality Profiles. [Online]. Available at:

http://www.who.int/whosis/mort/profiles/mort_amro_bra_brazil.pdf

WHOSIS, US. (2002). US Mortality Profiles. [Online]. Available at: http://www.who.int/whosis/mort/profiles/mort_amro_usa_unitedstatesofamerica.pdf).

About the Author

*Sandra Nuñez, **B.A., M.A.,*** enjoys being a freelance writer and traveling to distant lands. She grew up in Imperial Valley, California, and credits her sensitivity of cultural competence to this experience. Her degrees from the University of California Irvine, and the University of California Los Angeles, with majors in Anthropology, Social Science, and Latin American Studies, she credits to Divine Providence and her husband, Joe. She has collaborated in several books, including *Encyclopedia of Multicultural Psychology*, and *Latina/o Healing Practices: Mestizo and Indigenous Perspectives*. She lives in southern California. Her URL website address is: www.soulfulwriting.com Her email address is sandranunez222@yahoo.com

To order copies of

Brazil's Soulful Medicine,

please call (877) BUY-BOOK;

visit www.BuyBooksOnTheWeb.com;

or send $14.95 (plus $4.50 shipping and handling)

per book to

Infinity Publishing

1094 New DeHaven Street, Suite 100

West Conshohocken, PA 19428

Made in United States
Troutdale, OR
11/03/2026

56845232R00128